100 Days of Keto

by Laurie WJN

ISBN 9781728715711

Introduction

Both my husband and I are overweight, and not just a little overweight. My daughter asked us to please try the Keto diet. I was very skeptical, but at her insistence we gave it a try. I have been blogging my dieting experience each day, but I realized not everyone has the time to scroll through 100 individual daily blogs, so I have put all of my daily posts together in this book.

This book is NOT full of Keto diet plans, recipes or advice. While there may be some recipes and I might share what I have learned through doing some research this book is just me, sharing my personal experience. I know when I start something new, especially something like a diet; I want to hear from other people who have tried it. What worked? What didn't? What would you do differently? I am sharing my experience so that others can hear our story and decide for themselves if Keto is a good choice.

Our Keto Journey

Day 1-
Its no secret, my hubby and I are overweight. Although I have been overweight most of my adult life, I was much thinner when I met my hubby ten years ago.

Weight is insidious; it creeps up when you aren't paying attention. My hubby loves food, especially the unhealthy kind. Having lots of sweet treats around the house makes it nearly impossible to resist. My hubby is also a generous and loving person, so when I would crave salty potato chips he would oblige me by running up to the store and getting not one BIG bag, but usually two. Again, as I have said, it's nearly impossible for me to resist goodies when they are right in front of me. Its pretty easy to see how the past ten years have added up to quite a few additional pounds.

It wasn't just the food we are both couch potatoes. We honestly love to just snuggle on the couch and watch T.V. together. I used to jog and go workout and go hiking, I even completed a half marathon, but somehow over time it just seemed easier to stay home with Peter. Slowly but surely I began to exercise less and I packed on even more pounds.

Generally I don't give much thought to my weight, I tend to rely on cognitive dissonance, I know I am overweight but I just don't really see it most days. I look in the mirror and I know I am fat, but I just ignore it. Of course there are some moments when even I cannot ignore it. Buying a bathing suit is an uncomfortable reality, but lets be fair ladies, even when we are thin its uncomfortable to try on bathing suits. They tend to show off every flaw. Flying on a plane is another one of those uncomfortable realities. Acknowledging that the seatbelt is extended to its full length is scary; no one wants the embarrassment of asking for a seatbelt extender.

Obviously it is time to lose some weight. Although I am not a fan of dieting in general because they usually are not effective long term and I hate to support the multibillion dollar diet industry built on lies, my daughter was urging my husband and I to try the Keto diet, at least for a month or two to help kick start our weight loss. I was/am skeptical. I did lots of research and found lots of glowing endorsements for Keto as an effective weight loss technique, there is still little evidence that it a truly sustainable lifestyle. Despite all of this I did not find evidence that Keto actually causes any harm so we decided to try it.

Today is day 1 of our Keto journey. Realistically I would love to lose 100 pounds, and I am pretty sure that would be a fair goal for my chubby hubby too. The big key to this whole Keto diet is that without carbs, your body will actually begin to burn fat. This sounds good - I have plenty to burn.

The diet itself feels very antithetical to any diet plan I had every heard of. On Keto you are allowed, even encouraged to eat fat. Yes FAT: butter, cream, bacon, etc. Eating this fat along with protein and low carb produce while not eating any foods high in carbs (bread, grains, cereals, pasta) and avoiding foods high in sugar (again carbs) causes a phenomenon in your body called ketosis which actually encourages your body to burn fat for energy.

My first day I had my coffee and I still used my creamer even though it does have some carbs, but when it runs out I will transition to using heavy cream in my coffee, and for me I will add a drop of vanilla for flavor. I had some egg salad for lunch, a handful of almonds for a snack and then when my hubby got home we both had a filet and some beautiful asparagus for dinner. We both felt full and happy after dinner. So far so good.

I am not sure if this Keto diet will work, but I know I do need to get more active and get some of these pounds off. I want to be healthy to play with my grandson and do all the traveling that I have planned so I guess the Keto diet can be a good first step. I will continue to blog my journey so you all can follow along with me.

Day 2
I have been so overwhelmed with positive messages of support after posting my Day 1 blog. It is only Day 2 but so far so good. In the morning I had my coffee (still with regular creamer until is runs out) but even usual daily routines can be affected when counting carbs. My 'Fiber Choice" supplements have 7 carbs – yikes! I guess I will have to look for some fiber pills without carbs.

For breakfast today I made myself two scrambled eggs with some cheese. I ate my breakfast late so I managed to just have an Atkins bar for a quick lunch before heading out to work. I really worked hard at increasing my amount of water, which is hard for me as I am not a natural water drinker so I do have to push myself. For dinner I made myself a piece of fish with some lemon pepper and butter. Just a quick side note, I was not paying attention and went to shake a little of the lemon pepper but apparently I had opened the larger side so a huge pile of lemony pepper covered my fish, I had to shake it off and rise the pan quickly, but after cooking it came out great. I also made myself some yummy slices of zucchini that I tossed in some olive oil and spices and then covered with Parmesan. That was delicious and I will definitely make that again. I really have not been hungry so far.

My hubby brought himself a hamburger patty and a couple cheese sticks to work, and he had to work late so when he got home he made himself a steak for dinner. I did offer to make him some veggies but he said he was fine with just his steak (which sounded like a bad idea to me). I am always trying to get my hubby to eat more veggies.

Later in the evening I decided to splurge on a small glass of dry red wine, which according to my research does not have a lot of carbs. When Peter began to have his late night snack cravings I gave him a yummy Atkins candy bar that I had bought and since I had splurged on the wine I did not have one of the candy bars myself, but I did take a bit and it was good. According to the package it has only 2 net carbs. I know Peter has a sweet tooth so for him to be successful

on this diet I knew I had to be prepared with some snacks that he
was allowed to have.

I have not yet experienced any of the "Keto Flu" symptoms that
people talk about and honestly I am doing okay with my carb free
lifestyle right now. Watching TV is hard though, there are so many
commercials with chips and pizza and all kinds of goodies that we
can't/shouldn't have.

There is a pizza place near us that has cauliflower crust pizza so we
might have to have a date night this weekend and see if that Pizza
will suffice for Peter's pizza cravings (he loves pizza).

Now that we are getting out diet organized, our next step is to
increase our activity level. I am hoping to get Peter to come with me
to the YMCA tomorrow, but even if he doesn't want to go, I really
have to make myself go anyway. Keto will only work if I can
increase the number of calories I burn. My body won't start burning
fat unless it actually needs those calories from increased exercise.

Another benefit of going to the YMCA is that I can weigh myself.
We don't currently own a scale; our cheap old one broke and was
thrown away. I have never been a big fan of focusing on the exact
number on the scale, but in this case I do want to track my changes
over time on this diet so having a starting point and then doing
weekly checks of my progress are important to keep me motivated
(or at least that's wishful thinking on my part).

I am really struggling over the idea of sharing my actual weight.
This is extremely scary for any overweight person. To have people
actually know how much I weigh is terrifying, but it also can be a
powerful force for getting me to work hard at losing weight. I am
not sure if I am brave enough, but it is only a number after all.

Thanks again for all the encouragement and good wishes – they
really do help!

Day 3-
Our Keto adventure is continuing. I am still feeling full, but I really do miss some of my favorite carbs, especially at breakfast. No toast, no cereals, no oatmeal, no pancakes or waffles, so many of our typical breakfast foods contains huge amounts of carbs, even yogurt is banned because almost all of the yogurts contain lots of sugar. I will have to look up some recipes for Keto breakfast alternatives because I really can't see having eggs every single morning.

I have been keeping a food diary. I know that research proves folks who keep a food diary actually lose more weight. I am not really counting calories, that is just not in my personality and besides I hate math, but I can write down exactly what I am eating. This keeps me more accountable for what I eat.

Yesterday I was home all day so I found myself snacking more than usual. I started my day with coffee and a cheese stick. I had an Atkins bar for lunch. I snacked on some beef jerky and some pecans in the afternoon. For dinner I had a few bites of one of the hamburgers Peter made for his dinner while I was cooking mine. I sautéed some onions and garlic and then pan seared a piece of salmon, and I steamed some broccoli. I was so full I couldn't finish it all. After dinner Peter and I each had one small Atkins chocolate peanut butter cup while watching a movie we rented. (By the way – Game Night is hilarious).

I was busy doing chores so I was trying to be lazy and tell myself that I didn't need to go workout, but my daughter pushed me, so I put on my tennis shoes and headed to the YMCA. I really am out of shape, but I did manage to walk a steady pace for over 35 minutes and I was sweating. I brought my iPad and listened to an audible book as I was walking which helped to distract me and made the time pass more quickly. I think this is a good strategy. I know that it will take some time to get back into shape.

I did go and weight myself. I have gained even more weight than I thought so I really do need this diet and I hope it will help to kick start my new healthy lifestyle. And yes I am procrastinating here – I am still struggling with sharing my actual weight, but I know if I put that number out here, first of all, its just a number, it is not the sum total of my worth as a person. Secondly, that number is just a starting point of my journey – it does not hold any power over me. I now weigh 289 pounds. Ugh! I need to lose 100 pounds. I wish there was an easy button to push and it would be finished, but this will be a long journey.

Day 4-
Four days in and we're still going strong. I did come across some challenges, but was able to stay focused on and on track.

First, I went over to a friend's house in the morning, and everyone was enjoying mimosas and donuts. Yikes! I can't have either of those. It was hard being there and seeing everyone enjoying all those carbs. I decided to accept my friend's offer of a mimosa, but I asked him for only half a glass. I allowed myself two small sips so I wouldn't feel left out. I know that it is really important to maintain my diet, my body won't go into ketosis if I cheat, but I also know that allowing myself a small sip is important so I won't feel deprived. I also accepted the drink so I didn't have to feel awkward and tell everyone that I am on a diet. After my two small sips I put my glass down and continued to drink my water. I didn't even look at the donuts, which is tough because I really love donuts. Socializing with friends is great but it usually involves food, so it is important to be aware of the pitfalls.

Later in the day hubby and I met a friend to go see a movie, the latest new Marvel film Ant Man & the Wasp. Once again I was tempted, going to the movies is synonymous with eating popcorn, which is definitely NOT on the Keto diet. Just walking in the theatre and smelling all that yummy carb loaded popcorn, I could feel my mouth watering. Luckily I did plan ahead for the movie. I packed myself a container with some pecans and almonds. I was able to crunch and munch on a healthy alternative snack, and the movie was so good that I didn't even notice the lack of popcorn.

I was not able to make it to the YMCA because they close early on the weekends, but I did go out in the pool and do swim jogging for at least 15 minutes. It's not much but it is something. I also parked extremely far from the theatre entrance, and I refused a ride to my car, instead choosing the walk. I am hoping that each of these small changes will add up to big results.

Dinner tonight was a yummy piece of salmon and more of those delicious Parmesan zucchini chips that I made the other day. Peter really liked them too. I really have not been hungry at all. I am hoping that I will have the same successful results as so many others on this Keto diet have had, even with two small sips of a mimosa today.

I do think the key to maintaining this diet is to plan ahead, like having my own snacks packed for the movie. Planning and a positive attitude is the key to success.

Day 5
It's been almost a week and I am happy to report we are still going strong.

I started my day with just heavy cream in my coffee, I added some vanilla but I still missed the sweetness of my usual creamer.

After doing some work on my computer for a couple hours I made my way to the YMCA and I managed to walk on the treadmill for 40 minutes. I listened to an audiobook for distraction and it did help. I can't jog, after breaking my ankle twice it just hurts too much when I try to run at all, but I was pretty happy with walking on an incline for 40 minutes, even though my legs were pretty sore by the end. I know that getting back to exercise is a big part of this weight loss journey.

I didn't bother getting on the scale yet since its only been two days since I weighed my self at the YMCA, and weekly weight checks seems like a better option for tracking progress.

I was doing some reading and found out that only one third of US citizens are at a healthy weight – that means two thirds are overweight or obese. Peter and I are definitely not alone in our struggle for weight loss. I was also surprised to learn that only one third of all men and women between ages 25 and 64 workout regularly. I feel like those two pieces of information fit well together so I am even more committed to find time for exercise each day.

I am still not feeling hungry at all, but I do sure miss those carbs. I had a great lunch of tuna fish and then I headed out to a work meeting. They had lovely bowls of snacks for us at the meeting and I couldn't eat any of it, so I just stuck to drinking water. One of the things I have noticed is that I am not getting tired in the afternoons like I usually do. Without those sugar highs and lows I don't feel that afternoon lull that so often comes after eating.

After the meeting I went over to an open house event at my local democrat office and once again they had amazing snacks – nachos and beer, but I couldn't have any. I sipped on a diet soda and had fun even without the goodies. It is tempting to eat those carbs, I know how great they will taste to me, but I really do want to do my best effort on this diet and see if I can get some results.

Once I got home I warmed up two hot dogs that Peter had grilled a few days ago, and I had 5 strawberries.

Peter has not weighed himself yet, but I can tell that he is slimming down already. He has been great about packing lunches for work, usually a salad and a hamburger patty. He packs some Italian dressing and a couple cheese sticks to snack on when he get hungry.

Planning ahead and not giving in to temptations really are the key to staying on track.

Day 6 -
Day six and our weight loss journey continues. I spent more time at home so I had less temptations to deal with, but here's a pro tip – DO NOT got to the grocery store when you are hungry AND dieting. I picked up a bunch of great healthy alternatives for carbs and so far my favorite was cauliflower rice. I know you can easily make this

yourself if you have a food processor, but it comes in bags or even in some frozen varieties. I'll talk more about my cauliflower rice later.

Today was hard to be motivated to go to the YMCA. My legs were really sore from the walking the day before, but I didn't want to allow myself any excuses. After a quick morning meeting, I came home changed into my workout clothes and got back on the treadmill. I am still using an audiobook to help pass the time during my workout. I used to listen to high-energy music when I ran, to help get me pumped up, but my ankle will absolutely not let me run right now, at least not with all this weight. I am hoping that as I continue to lose weight and exercise that maybe I will be able to strengthen my ankle and I can once again do some running; to be fair my version of running has always been a slow jog but I do regularly sign up for 5K's. I managed 25 minutes of walking and then decided my calves and ankles would really appreciate me if I switched to a bicycle for the last 15 minutes of the workout.

For food today; I started my day with coffee, I made myself some egg salad for lunch, I had some raspberries and pecans for a snack, I had an Atkins bars in the late afternoon while I was out, and I came home and made myself some salmon and cauliflower rice for dinner, and I had a cheese stick and some almonds for an evening snack. Once again I was a little hungrier today, which is why I had a few snacks throughout the day.

I absolutely loved the cauliflower rice. Cauliflower has 5g per cup vs. 46g for a cup of brown rice. I wasn't sure how to cook it so I looked online and there are lots of ways to prepare it; microwave, oven, stove. I chose to pan fry about two cups. I used some butter for flavor and a bit of oil to help make sure the butter didn't burn as quickly. I added some garlic, salt, and pepper. It was so good – it was exactly the carb feeling I was missing. I am now a big fan.

Peter is still doing great on his diet too and he is looking good. We both talked about actually feeling better without sugar, although Peter had me cracking up talking about how he would have killed for a cinnamon roll. With all of the monsoon storms the mornings are cooler so I am planning to take Lexi on a walk tomorrow morning, just to add some variety to my workouts and because she is really tired of being cooped up on the house. Normally it is way to hot to take a dog on a walk during Phoenix summers, but monsoons cool it off just enough to make it possible.

Day 7-
Officially one week into our diet and things are still going well.

I did manage to get up early and take Lexi on a walk. It was already getting pretty warm, but we walked down to the park and back and the walk includes a pretty decent hill to climb down and up so that helps adds to the intensity of the walk. Our walk was only about 35 minutes, Lexi was looking pretty hot and tired so we came home and we both jumped into the pool where I did some swimming and water jogging for another 15 minutes. I am trying to make sure I mix up my workout routines so I keep moving but I don't get too bored.

I realized I haven't been using my fitbit and that might be a good way to encourage more exercise so I found it got it charged up and put it on. Burning more calories means losing more weight.

I only had some coffee for breakfast. I made myself a yummy lettuce & turkey wrap with some feta cheese and a little but of ranch. I rolled it up like a burrito and it was fantastic. I also had some cucumber with it.

After Peter came home we did some cooking together. I made some more of that pan-fried cauliflower rice and Peter loved it. He said "Oh my god, this is delicious, lets go get more of this, can we go to Costco and get like a 50 pound bag" Yeah I'm pretty sure he liked it. Peter had some chicken that we cooked in a pan with some beautiful pepper, and I made myself some shrimp scampi using some frozen shrimp I had gotten and some fresh garlic.

I know it is hard to restrict carbs, but there are so many great food choices without using a bunch of carbs. I felt so good about how well we were doing that I even splurged on a glass of red wine, which I found out only has 3.8 carbs. Yeah!

One full week and we are still on track!

Day 8 –
I started my day meeting a friend at Starbucks and was pleased to
discover that the Keto coffee recipe for Starbucks I had read online
was actually pretty yummy. I ordered a regular coffee with two shots
of sugar free vanilla syrup and real cream.

I will admit I was struggling with energy today, I think that infamous
Keto flu is to blame. I had read about it, and during this week I felt
great except for a little occasional dizziness, but it is always hard to
decipher if that is due to my diet or just one of the many joys of
menopause.

I did a few errands and came home, where I had a big lunch of
lettuce turkey wraps again, but today I added some avocado slices
with the feta cheese. It was so good. I also had some cucumber.

Feeling creatively inspired I worked on a few writing projects and
before I knew it, it after 4:00 and Peter had stopped at home to grab
something to eat before heading back to work for the evening. Peter
made himself a steak and again I bugged him about adding veggies
to his meals for healthy balance.

I snacked a little with a cheese stick, some beef jerky and then some
almonds. I was a little hungrier today. I decided to make myself a
big plate of grilled broccoli and cauliflower, which I had tossed in
some olive oil and spices with a bit of parmesan sprinkled on top. It
was delicious and definitely filled me up.

The only negative for the day was that lack of energy I felt. I
actually gave myself the day off from going to the YMCA. I think its
okay to give yourself a break once in awhile.

Now to share way too much information for those who are thinking
of doing the Keto diet and wondering how it will affect you, its time
to talk poop. I was wondering if there would be any changes with

this diet and I am happy to report that so far, I have not had any problems or issues.

Starting week two we are still on track and doing well. I hope I am losing weight, I can tell that Peter is.

Day 9 –
After over a week on our diet, I am excited to announce that I have lost 3 pounds!

It has only been 4 days since I weighed myself, so its not actually a full week of weight loss, but its still a good number. I do have to admit that while I'm proud of losing 3 pounds, I am just a tiny bit disappointed. After years of watching shows like Biggest Loser with their incredibly unhealthy and unrealistic weight loss amounts I was really hoping for some dramatic double digit number, but life isn't like a fake reality TV show and healthy weight loss is 1-2 pounds per week so I am actually ahead of the curve.

Our biggest accomplishment so far was staying on the diet – both Peter and I have done really well without sneaking any carbs. I think that is a big deal. And while I do look longingly at ads on TV with bread or chips, I honestly haven't felt deprived.

Today I started my day with some coffee. It was already too hot by 9:00am to take Lexi on a walk (I won't take her if it is over 90 degrees) so I did some housework, wrote my daily blog post and then a conference call for work. In the afternoon I headed over to the YMCA, where I decided to do a weigh in. I walked on the treadmill for 35 minutes and then did a few of the weight machines before finishing off with 10 minutes on one of the bicycles.

When I go home I made myself a salad with some feta cheese and a few bacon bits, and then I snacked on some almonds in the afternoon.

We had been talking about trying the Cauliflower Crust pizza so around 5:00 I texted Peter to see if he wanted to get pizza and he

answered right away. It was our celebration date night after our first
full week of Keto. The Pizza was so good, we honestly thought
maybe there was a mistake and they had given us a regular crust by
mistake. Cauliflower is the greatest! The crust was crunchy and
wonderful. Only 3.6 carbs per slice! What a perfect way to celebrate
and indulge, without actually going off our diet.

After such a positive first week and such a fun yummy celebration,
we are both energized and ready to keep going!

Day 10-
After a quick cup of coffee Lexi and I started the morning with a
nice long walk. Not only is it healthy exercise for me, but she really
appreciates the chance to smell every single tree and bush in my
little corner of Phoenix.

I came home and did some chores, and then Peter and I had fun
cooking breakfast together, although it was more like brunch to be
honest. He made me a fantastic bacon and cheese omelet, he made
himself a ham and chees omelet, and I sautéed some onions and
added them to some pan-fried cauliflower rice. It gave us the feeling
of potatoes on our plate without the carbs.

Weekends are good for getting housework done, so we spent a few
hours cleaning, and then I went out canvassing for some great local
candidates. Not only am I helping our democracy but I am getting
some exercise too.

Afterward I came home and we finally made the cauliflower version
of mac-n-cheese that I had been promising him. It was delicious, but
sadly it does not actually taste like macaroni. The cheese was gooey
and creamy, and we might have added a bit extra, but with only 29
total carbs in an entire head of cauliflower I could technically eat the
entire pan and not be over on my daily carbs, this is a great healthy
option.

Here is the recipe that I found online, although it says bake for 15
minutes and we found it needs at least 25 minutes to really melt well

and get a slightly crispy crust on top. We just used our hand to break up the florets and that seemed to work really well.

Cauliflower Mac N Cheese
1 large head of cauliflower chopped into florets. Cook that in microwave for about 5 minutes or until soft. Place in a 9x9 oven dish.

For the cheese sauce:
1 cup heavy cream
2 oz. cream cheese
1 cup cheddar cheese
2 tsp. spicy mustard
2 tsp. garlic powder

15 minutes at 375

I have been wearing my fitbit and even with a walk in the morning and canvassing in the afternoon, I still only managed a little over 7,000 steps so I still have to increase my exercise if I want to reach the 10,000 steps every day recommended by the American Heart Association.

Each day we are getting closer to our goals so I know its worth it, and it really helps that Peter and I are doing this together. Having support at home really does make all the difference for me, it gives me the reinforcement I need to stick with it.

Day 11-
Peter and I got up and started our day with a visit to the YMCA. I am super excited to report that I have lost 7 pounds so far since weighing myself on Day 3. That's right – I have lost one pound per day! I know that I am able to lose a larger amount right now because I have a lot more to lose than some folks, but I am really happy with my progress so far. I still have a really long way to go, but I am on the right track.

At the YMCA Peter swam and met his personal goal, and I walked
on the treadmill for 25 minutes and then finished on a bicycle for a
little over 10 minutes. We both decided to have a lazy day after our
YMCA visit so after a few quick household chores Peter spent some
time playing his video games and I spent some time reading and
writing.

For lunch I ate some of the leftover cauliflower mac-n-cheese dish. I
had some snacks throughout the afternoon, some almonds and a
cheese stick. At dinner I made myself some cauliflower rice and
some shrimp that I pan-fried in butter. I am trying to make sure that I
have enough fat in my diet.

I was really craving something to munch on in the evening. I tried a
cheese stick, but it just didn't work. I grabbed a handful of pecans
and it was okay but I was really missing being able to crunch on a
cracker or something.

Day 12 –
Lexi and I had a nice morning walk today, but it was already getting
hot quickly so we came home after only a mile. Phoenix summers
are really hard for outdoor exercise of any kind. I know Lexi was
hot and tired because the minute we walked into the nice air-
conditioned house she plopped down on the tile floor and spread out,
just enjoying the feel of the cool stone.

My new challenge today was eating out. I had made plans with my
amazing friend Susan. I have know her for more than 30 years and
although she lives on the other side of town, we always manage to
find time to see each other every few months to get together for
some girl time and catch up on life. Usually this involves a meal.
We made plans to meet for lunch and the restaurant had a great salad
bar so I was all set. I just had to avoid any croutons or crackers and
skip the carrots and I had a nice low carb lunch. After finishing our
salads, Susan had some of the self-serve ice cream. She was sweet
and asked me, "You don't mind do you? Will this be hard if I have
this?" but honestly it wasn't hard. I had grabbed some walnuts to
much on and it was fine.

I am not sure that I have some great reserve of will power, but I know that I am working towards my goal. I want to be thinner and healthier so I can comfortably travel to all the great places I hope to visit and I want to have the energy to enjoy playing with my amazing beautiful grandchild. Making healthy choices about my food will get me closer to those goals.

Susan and I talked about the diet and I shared how we were doing. We both commiserated on how much harder it is to lose weight once you are in menopause, so she was interested in how I was doing on the Keto diet. I feel like we're doing great staying on track, but Peter and I are not letting this diet take over our lives, we are just trying hard to be more aware of food choices. I have been reading food labels as I shop, looking at the number of carbs. I have checked the amount of carbs online when I am not sure, so we can make good decisions and still stay within our goals.

I know some people are extremely serious about their Keto diets; carefully counting every single carb and something called macros. According to Google, "The term "macros" is short for MACRONUTRIENTS in the context of nutrition and the Keto diet. Macronutrients are the energy-giving components of food that fuels our body. They include carbohydrates, protein, and fat; this is where your dietary calories come from." Basically some people carefully count the percentages of fats, proteins and carbs for everything they eat. Peter and I are looking at foods and trying to make good choices, but we certainly aren't going around with a calculator checking on what percentage of protein vs. fat is in each item we eat. If we tried to do that this diet would already have been over for both of us. We just aren't that kind of people. We are both just giving a lot more thought to what we eat. Peter explained that having limited choices is helping him to eat less and I would agree, plus I do think I had a carb heavy diet before so this is a big change for my body.

We did have an oops moment at dinner. I asked what vegetable he wanted, and Peter said he wanted lima beans with his meal. He made himself a steak and I had a piece of salmon and I prepared the lima beans. After serving both of us, I started thinking about lima beans so I looked up the total carbs and whoops, there are 39 carbs in a cup. We hadn't eaten too many, so we both felt like we had half a cup or less. I knew that corn and potatoes were high in carbs, but all types of beans and legumes are also really high in carbs. Oh well, we won't make that mistake again and I think we both were able to still stay under our daily goal of less than 25 total carbs.

Day 13 –
Yes! Costco for the win! While picking up some almonds and pecans I found amazing Parmesan Cheese Crisps. They have only one carb per serving, so when I have that need for something to crunch I can grab a few of these.

Almost 2 weeks into our diet and we are still doing well. It has surprised me how easy it has actually been to stay on our diet. Buying some of the Keto 'cheater foods' like the crisps has helped.

I started my day off with a Starbucks 'Keto' coffee (2 shots of sugar free vanilla and heavy cream). After a busy morning I came home and had some tuna for lunch. I snacked on some of the Cheese Crisps and they were great. They have a great crunch but they are a little tangy.

Peter came home and we made dinner. He cooked us both a small filet and a couple scallops and I made some oven-roasted asparagus. I wound up giving my scallops to Peter.

After dinner I headed out to the YMCA and got on the treadmill for just over 40 minutes. My ankle was getting sore, but I really wanted to finish a full 40 minutes. After working out I stepped on the scale. I know that I had said I would only weigh myself once a week, but I was curious how I was doing and I am happy to report that I lost another pound, so that's 8 pounds total in the two weeks. I still have a long way to go but I am feeling really encouraged by my results so far.

Day 14-

We have made it officially two weeks into our diet so far.

I had another busy day, which started with another restaurant challenge; a breakfast meeting. The only good Keto option for breakfast was eggs with bacon or sausage. I do like eggs and bacon, but I am struggling with the lack of variety for breakfast. I think this has been one of the hardest things for me on this Keto diet.

After my morning meeting I did some errands and came home, where I managed to do a few chores and work on some writing projects. I made myself a nice salad for lunch with lettuce, a whole bunch of cucumber, some feta cheese, and some pumpkin seeds for extra flavor and crunch.

I had a handful of the crisps and a cup of almonds as a snack in the afternoon, and then Peter and I ran out to a candidate forum event in the evening. It was late when we headed home so I actually skipped dinner, but I did eat a quick yummy nut bar I had gotten at Costco. Choosing to eat the nut bar, I wanted to make sure that I was correctly counting my carbs. There is a difference between total carbs and net carbs. In this nut bar for example there are 14 total grams of carbs, but there are 7 grams of dietary fiber so you can subtract the fiber from the total to get only 7 net carbs in one bar.

According to most of the sources I have read you can have up to 50 total carbs or up to 20-25 net carbs per day.

Total carbohydrates – Dietary Fiber = Net Carbs

I spent some time reading more sources about Keto, including an inspiring story by a woman who has lost over 100 pounds on Keto and has continued to keep the weight off for three years now.

Since we are two weeks into this diet, I decided it was time to learn a bit more. Apparently Peter and I are doing something called 'Lazy Keto' which is totally not surprising. Basically this is just folks like us who are not worrying about exact percentages, we are just trying to keep our daily carbs under 20 grams.

The non-lazy version of the diet is folks who make sure their diet percentages of fats, proteins and carbs are carefully balanced. I did find an online 'keto calculator' and after entering some info here is my ideal percentage, or as Keto folks describe, these are my macros.

I did not have the chance to make it to the YMCA today, so I will definitely have to make time to go tomorrow.

Peter and I are both sticking with this diet and we are seeing results. There are still moments when I really do miss some of my favorite carb-loaded foods, but I know we are working toward our goals. We both have talked about the fact that we have not felt hungry at all; the only real challenge is the limited choice of foods that we can eat. This Keto diet isn't always easy, but we are both doing a great job of sticking with it so far.

Day 15 –
We have noticed something interesting happening, both Peter and I are eating less. We are eating less and not feeling hungry.

After a morning coffee, Peter made bacon and eggs for us. We ate around 10:00 and this actually kept me full until having a snack of some almonds in the afternoon. I had a meeting in the evening so I basically skipped dinner and I honestly did not feel hungry. I cam home and had a couple cheese sticks and Peter and I both had an Atkins peanut butter cup candy while watching TV.

I really wish there were some better low carb options for breakfast. Right now our only choice has been eggs. I am going to do some research to find some other breakfast choices. There are so many great options for lunch and dinner, and I feel really good about the snack choices we have been using like almonds, pecans, beef jerky, cheese sticks and those cheese crisps. Even those silly Atkins fake candies are great when we really want a goodie (although they are not truly Keto, the Atkins diet is much higher in protein).

I have been really consistent making it to the YMCA at least every other day. The mornings have been hotter this past week, so I can't do any walks with Lexi right now.

I think this is one of the really challenging times in our diet because the newness has worn off and we have to buckle down and continue to stay on track. I really struggle with monotony so I need to spend some time getting creative and finding new and interesting food options that are Keto friendly.

Another challenge for me has been the personal commitment I made to write this blog each day. I decided to write this in the hopes that I can encourage other people who might be considering this diet, and so that I can honestly share how things are going for us. It is hard to always find the time to get each daily post written and shared online. I want to continue to blog daily at least for the first month of our diet, but hopefully I can continue to share our story for as long as we stay on Keto. I want to make sure I am not getting boring and just repeating my daily food diary, but that I am actually sharing useful information.

As we enter our third week of dieting I am feeling encouraged, and I have every confidence we will keep going.

Day 16-
I have been surprised and quite frankly amazed at how many people have heard of or are currently doing the Keto diet. After feeling frustrated yesterday with our limited food choices so far, I have been focused on learning more about Keto recipes.

After starting my day with coffee I got busy with work and then grabbed one of my low carb nut bars for a quick breakfast snack.

Later I chopped up some leftover chicken and added 1 strip of chopped bacon, some chopped pecans for flavor & crunch, a handful of broccoli rice and some mayonnaise for a super yummy chicken salad. Peter tried it and said it was delicious. There are so many fun options to add into the food that are still Keto friendly.

I did not make it to the YMCA today. I am still averaging at least every other day, but I would like to get to the point where I am working out daily. Some days there is just too much going on and I simply run out of time. I am just not the kind of person who wakes up early to go workout and I probably never will be. One of the challenges I have in working out is that I get extremely sweaty when I workout, so I have to plan time to take a shower which means a trip to workout has to happen at least 2 hours before I need to go somewhere. So I ran out of time to get to the Y and still have time for a shower before our evening plans

In the evening we went to visit some friends. It was another important test of our Keto diet resolve. Our friends had managed to make a perfect meal for our diet; they grilled vegetables in foil packets with some delicious chicken. We had a salad and then the chicken and veggies, so I felt okay actually having two glasses of wine, feeling reasonably confident that I was still under my carb limit. Peter did break down and have a beer so he was probably over his carbs just a bit.   We joked and teased with our friends that we were so glad that hadn't planned spaghetti. It does bring up an issue for dieting – making sure friends and family know that you have a limited diet.

It is pretty incredible that we have been doing so well for 16 days now, and hopefully the scale will reflect all of our hard work.

Day 17-
Happy to report we made it to the YMCA today, I have been able to maintain at least every other day since starting the diet. I am sure that is part of why I am doing well losing weight, and the super exciting news is that I have lost even more. So far I have lost about 12 pounds! That's a really great start but we have a long way to go.

I started the day with some coffee and I grabbed a quick Atkins bar because I was late to a meeting. After I got home I made myself some zucchini with Parmesan. It is super easy, just slice the zucchini and toss with some olive oil and spices, then top with some Parmesan and bake for about 10 minutes.

We headed out to the YMCA and then went over to a party to celebrate a friend's graduation. Once again we had to be careful to make good #Keto choices. They had yummy shredded pork and several big bowls of potato salad, macaroni salad and coleslaw, most of which we couldn't have. Choosing to have some pork without the bun was a simple way to keep Keto.

After leaving the party we splurged again on some cauliflower crust pizza and I even had a beer. Miller Lite has only 3.2 carbs and sometimes you just need a beer with your pizza.

It is really encouraging to see such incredible results for all of our hard work; it helps give us the motivation to keep working hard and making good choices.

Day 18 –
I started my day with my usual coffee and then made myself some scrambled eggs, with some leftover bacon. I really do like ot eat bacon and eggs, just not every morning. I did find a recipe for cauliflower toast, but I haven't had a chance to try it yet.

After taking some time to write and share my blog I headed out to go volunteer at a voter registration event for the morning.

Once I got home spent some time surfing through social media, and tried to give myself a reason to no go workout. I'm tired, I woke up really early, I'm sore, I just want a day off, I had a litany of excuses in my head, but I made myself go anyway.

I walked for almost 45 minutes on the treadmill and when I came home I was a sweaty mess, so Peter and I went swimming in our pool to cool off. I know that pushing myself to go to the YMCA even when I don't feel like it is going to get me back to the level of fitness where I want to be, but it is so hard. I really was looking for any excuse to stay home, but I am really glad I forced myself to get moving.

I snacked on some Crisps and then in the evening I made myself some shrimp and cauliflower rice, Peter made a steak, and I bugged him to make sure he also had a vegetable, so he steamed some broccoli, which he shared with me. It was so good.

I have a lot going on this week, but I am going to try to fit a trip to the YMCA in every single day if I can. It is supposed to be really hot, so I don't think Lexi and I will be doing any walks this week, but we are dog-sitting a cute puppy for a friend so she will be busy playing with Diggity Dog.

This week's goal is to stay motivated to exercise and to stay on track with our diet.

Day 19 –
So I'm totally doing what I said I shouldn't do and I'm weighing myself daily, so naturally I have not lost anything for the past two days and I'm feeling frustrated. I know that all diets will have peaks and valleys as my body adjusts to this new normal. I guess this is even more reason why I need to workout daily to help my metabolism and burn all this fat I have.

Once again I began my day with just some coffee and later in the morning I had a small snack of some pecans. I am trying to concentrate on drinking more water to make sure I am adequately hydrated, and as my daughter likes to remind me, sometimes you might feel hungry when you are actually just thirsty.

I went early to the YMCA and I did 20 minutes on the stationary bicycle and then 25 more minutes on the treadmill. My ankle has been getting a little sore when I do the treadmill for too long so I am trying to make sure and keep variety. I also make sure to warm up carefully with some stretches and some ankle circles to help loosen those stiff joints.

I have been writing my blog each day in a word document and then pasting each entry onto my blog, along with added pictures. I have already written 29 pages so far. I might actually think about releasing this whole story as an eBook in the future. I'm not really sure, but it is an idea to consider. I know that many family and friends have commented that they are reading my posts and several people have talked about doing a similar diet. If my experiences could help other people that would be great. I read a few stories from people who have lost weight on the Keto diet and I thought it was helpful to hear about their experience as I started my diet.

I know some people get angry when someone says, "I forgot to eat". Like how could you ever forget to eat? But today I got so busy doing work that I looked up and realized it was almost 2:00 and I hadn't really eaten anything, I also realized I was hungry so I headed to the kitchen. I used some leftover rotisserie chicken, which I cup up and then added some pecans, one cut up cheese stick and a small amount of cauliflower rice and mixed with mayonnaise, which came out as a super yummy chicken salad. I really like food with a variety of texture and this was crunchy and chewy and really tasted great; it filled me up.

I do know that some people on the Keto diet do restrict their food intake to a certain eating window of time, like 10:00am-6:00pm or 12:00 to 8:00pm. For me, since there are so few breakfast options I have found myself skipping breakfast, but it is not an intentional diet strategy. There is so much information out there are dieting approaches, and quite frankly most of them are not based on sound science, so I am hesitant to follow them.

There is some great research on the Keto diet. I easily found two recent articles from Harvard and National Institutes of Health supporting the Keto diet as an effective means of weight loss (click on the links to read each one).

From Harvard:
https://www.health.harvard.edu/blog/ketogenic-diet-is-the-ultimate-low-carb-diet-good-for-you-2017072712089

From N.I.H:
https://www.ncbi.nlm.nih.gov/pmc/articles/PMC2716748/

I did not find the same glowing endorsements for Intermittent fasting as a dieting approach, but there does seem to be some evidence suggesting fasting can be an effective weight management tool.

According to the popular Keto website ruled.me.com,

There are a few approaches when it comes to intermittent fasting.

- **Skipped meals**. This is when you skip over a meal to induce extra time of fasting. Usually people choose breakfast, but others prefer to skip lunch.
- **Eating windows**. Usually this condenses your entire macronutrient intake between a 4 and 7 hour window. The rest of the time you are in a fasting state.
- **24-48 hour cleanse**. This is where you go into extended fasting periods, and do not eat for 1-2 days.

I am not particularly in favor of any of these methods, but the website does discuss how one of these options might help if you have stalled in your weight loss. I don't believe I'm there yet, but I have always believed that it is a good idea to restrict eating after 7:00pm or 8:00pm because late eating is simply calories that are not effectively burned off. Somehow I envision eating and then going to sleep with all those pesky little calories rushing straight to my hips and thighs.

For now just choosing healthy Keto foods and trying to incorporate healthy exercise routines into my lifestyle are more than enough for me.

For dinner, I was actually still feeling a little full from lunch so I cut up a zucchini and made more of those delicious baked zucchini and Parmesan chips. It was perfect.

I have been finding some fun Keto recipes online, but right now it is so hot out, and the last thing I really feel like doing is a bunch of cooking in a hot kitchen. Phoenix summer can be brutal like that. I looked online at a spiralizer, and I may decide to get one. Having more healthy food options sounds like a great thing.

For now we are continuing to do really well maintaining our Keto diet and making good choices with out food, even if we still longingly dream about chips and donuts.

Day 20 –
I decided that I needed to try a new recipe so this morning I made myself some Keto Cauliflower toast.

Here is the link for the recipe
https://www.delish.com/cooking/recipes/a50033/cauliflower-toast-recipe/
It was a little strange at first, I tried to grate the cauliflower on the small grate side – this does not work. When I used the larger shred size it worked perfectly and soon I had a big pile of mush. The recipe didn't say if it needed to be covered in the microwave so I left it uncovered. I did put a paper towel in the bottom of the bowl to help squish out liquid, but after 8 minutes there wasn't much liquid to squish out. The recipe suggests making the piles into toast shapes and as you can see I failed completely, but I popped them into the oven for 20 minutes and they actually looked okay but they did NOT come off the tin foil. What I was able to peel/scrape up actually tasted pretty good. I am well known for Pinterest fails. The recipe actually said use parchment paper, and at the very least I should have used cooking spray on the foil. Second, I may have used a bit more cheese than the recipe called for so that might have added to the stickiness. Overall it tasted okay so I might try again, now that I know what I am doing.

I do feel like that kitchen disaster was an omen for the rest of my day. I really wanted to go workout, but I had a bunch of stuff I needed to get done for work, and I had an early afternoon appointment with a client for work, so I basically ran out of time. Then I forgot to pack some healthy snacks, so I was starting to get hungry. After work I went straight to an evening commitment I had without stopping to eat anything.

I spent the evening volunteering making phone calls for a candidate that I support and they had a whole table of snacks but there was not one single item on the whole table that I could have. It was full of cookies, crackers, chips, candy, etc. I would have killed for just a few almonds. I dutifully drank my water but by the time I got home I was ravenous. I hate to eat really late so I tried to just grab a snack, but after two cheese sticks I was still hungry so I tried a small handful of almonds. That didn't really work so I grabbed the bag of crisps and ate about 10 of those. At that point I'm not sure if I was still hungry or just frustrated and hangry, but I resorted to a spoonful of natural peanut butter as my comfort food. When I went to bed I was really frustrated with myself. I think I can use my failures as a good lesson in what NOT to do. First – plan ahead and be prepared with healthy snacks that I CAN eat. Secondly, don't skip meals because it makes you much too hungry later. Third, and most importantly – it's okay to make mistakes. Messing up is not a big deal, just focus and get back on track.

Here's hoping tomorrow is a much more successful day!

Day 21 –
I'm not sure which is harder staying on this diet or having the discipline to do a blog post every day. I am also trying to write down a food journal each day so I can see what I am eating.

According to an article from realsimple.com

Writing down what you eat helps you take a critical look at your food habits and make healthy changes. Here are some tips.

- Record everything you eat and drink immediately.

- Note what you're doing while you're eating—driving, watching TV, etc.

- Describe how you felt while you ate: angry, sad, happy, nervous, starving, bored?

- Be honest. It's a journal, not a newsletter, and no one has to see it but you.

- At the end of each day, examine how your emotions affected your eating.

I am not writing down food immediately, but I try to make sure to write it down as soon as I can. This just feels like another level of accountability to help keep me eating healthy. According to Livestrong.com keeping a food journal has four main benefits; accountability, eating balanced meals, success attaining goals, and connecting food to feelings.

A big part of overeating is equating food to feelings. I actually am opposite from most people, I do eat out of boredom sometimes, but generally when I am angry, sad or upset I tend to eat a lot less. Understanding when and why you are eating is an important step in changing negative habits.

Today I started with my coffee. We are using the sugar free version of creamer since it has fewer carbs, only like two total carbs for a serving. After the mistakes of yesterday I want to make better food decisions today so I made myself some scrambled eggs with one piece of crumbled bacon and some shredded cheddar cheese.

I made it to the YMCA in the morning so I had plenty of time to get home and showered before working this afternoon. I jumped on the stationary bicycle for 10 minutes then I did the treadmill for 35 minutes.

We have officially been on this diet for three weeks now and….
Drum roll please….I have lost of total of 13 pounds!!! It is a
great feeling when the weight bar slides to the right.

Yeah! That is really encouraging and that is the kind of news that
keeps me motivated.

I had to rush out to work in the afternoon, but this time I also
brought a couple cheese sticks and one of those yummy nut bars so I
wouldn't get too hungry.

For dinner I made some broccoli rice for both of us, Peter had a
steak, which he enjoyed with fresh mushrooms, and I had a lovely
piece of salmon.

Feeling really good about my progress so far, I decided to celebrate
and splurge my carbs on a glass of red wine.

Three weeks and we are still on track – that really is something to
celebrate

Day 22 –
Starting our fourth week of Keto and I am excited about our progress
so far, but it is hard to see that long-term goal yet. Losing 13 pounds
is a fantastic accomplishment, but we both have such a long way to
go.

I guess the old adage of not seeing the forest for the trees applies
here.

I should try the technique they used on Biggest Loser, and get 13
pounds of something to hold and see how much that really is. I think
it could be a good motivator. Maybe when I go to the YMCA I can
pick up a 10 pounds weight.

When I get overwhelmed at the amount of weight we need to lose I
think that's a good time to use the mantra of addiction folks, just one
day at a time.

Peter finally weighed himself and WOW he has lost 23 pounds!
Guys always seem to lose weight faster than women.

So today I started with my usual cup of coffee. I had a few pecans in
the morning and then I had leftover salmon and a big salad for lunch.
I made it over to the YMCA and did 35 minute on the treadmill. It
was so hot out that I was sweaty before I even started working out.

When Peter got home we decided to be brave and try to make the
Keto Chicken Enchilada recipe that two different friends had shared
with me because they knew I was doing Keto.

https://www.facebook.com/KetoDailyRecipes/videos/204369566875
621/

First I made up the Chicken mix, but I used half a small can of green
enchilada sauce and I checked it has zero carbs. I also mixed in just a
teaspoon of sour cream to add some creaminess to the mixture.

This time I used parchment paper and put a handful of shredded
cheese into four piles that I smoothed out to a size that I thought
looked good.

We baked them for the 7 minutes that the recipe said and they came
out perfect.

We put the mixture on one side of the cheese and Peter helped to roll
each one.

They looked awesome. I put a small amount of sour cream on mine,
but Peter added even more of the green enchilada sauce and sour
cream on his.

We had fun making these together and we both agreed we would
definitely make them again.

I have decided to get a Keto cookbook so we can try even more
recipes and find some things that we both like.

Day 23 –
As we continue our fourth official week on Keto I have been doing
more research on the diet. Our lazy version of Keto has been very
effective for us so far. It does seem slightly ironic that doing
something in a lazy way can be effective, but you can't argue with
results.

Looking at a bunch of Keto websites, many of them offer 14 day or
30 day meal plans. I have never been the kind of person who can
follow one of those. Some people thrive on the structure of being
told exactly what to eat and when, but I usually feel suffocated by it
and quite often I find myself doing the exact opposite. I do think that
says a lot about my personality in general, but it is clear these meal
plans are not going to work for me.

I decided to order a couple Keto cookbooks; hopefully we
will continue to find a variety of interesting Keto recipes that Peter
and I can do together. The book that was most recommended on
some Keto Facebook groups was *Keto Clarity* by Jimmy Moore.

Several people also suggested *Keto Living Day By Day*. Since I had
a gift card I earned doing some market research I decided to splurge
and order both, as well as the spiralizer that folks recommended. It
seemed like a great use of my gift card.

I made myself some scrambled eggs and cheese for breakfast. I made
a big bowl of chicken salad for lunch; with plenty leftover because
Peter called and said he forgot his lunch today so he said he would
be starving when he gets home.

Today was a good day to catch up on small chores around the house
that I really needed to do.

My car has been struggling in the Arizona heat and I have had a lot
going on in the past few weeks and I decided that I needed to take a
day of rest and I skipped going to the Y today. I have an early
morning car appointment tomorrow so I might even walk down to

the Y while they work on my car, giving me an extra bonus. According to Google Maps its only .8 miles, but the big challenge will be walking in the heat. I will have to make sure to hydrate well – wish me luck. I don't feel guilty for skipping today because that sounds like a double workout for tomorrow. I do think it's important to take a day off once in awhile, just to rest and relax, especially where there is a lot going on in your life.

I was amazed that later in the evening when I already received part of my Amazon order. Technology is amazing. On a side note, I just love ordering from Amazon – it always feels like Christmas when you get to open a package, even if its something you order for yourself, even when its something not very exciting like allergy medicine, it is always a fun to open a package. The only main drawback is all the cardboard and packaging.

Anyway – I had ordered the Pork Rinds because several Keto websites and Facebook groups mentioned them.

I sat down and started looking through the new cookbook and marking several of the recipes that I want to make. It was interesting because several of the recipes used group up pork rinds, as a kind of breading so I think those will come in handy.
 The cookbook cover says it has 130 'deceptively simple recipes' and I do like that each recipe lists the Keto info for each one, with amount of carbs, fats, proteins and calories. I am looking forward to more variety in our meals; although we have been successful so far I always think its good to try new things.

Day 24 –
My YMCA adventure this morning was challenging but in a good way. I dropped off the car and with my headphones on and a bottle of water in my hand I headed over to the Y. According to Google it was .8 miles and luckily there was some shade along the walk, since it was already over 90 degrees before 9am.

Once at the Y, I spent about 20 minutes on the bicycle and then did several of the weight machines, focusing on arms. I refilled my water bottle, sat for a few minutes answering some family text messages, and then I began the very warm walk back to the car shop. I was grateful to sit in the air conditioning while I waited for another 45 minutes for my car to finish. I was really starting to get hungry so I was bummed that I didn't have a Keto friendly snack with me. When they finished with my car I still had a couple errands to finish so I ate a few of the pecans I had in my purse but was still hungry so I decided to stop at McDonalds and got one cheeseburger. I made sure to ask for no ketchup. I threw away the bun and just ate the hamburger patty so I know that was Keto friendly. It was the perfect amount so I didn't feel hungry.

I did a few more errands, stopped by my work to drop off some files and then headed home. I was feeling really tired and I think that was due to the heat. I had the leftover chicken salad and then decided to go for a quick swim to cool off.

After finishing a few chores I made myself some cauliflower rice and shrimp for dinner. I was hoping to have some other veggies with it, but we didn't have any good options available. I need to get more vegetables when I go to the store this week.

Peter got home a few hours later and we went outside to swim. We began talking about our dieting experience so far. We still long for carb loaded goodies, I want starches - chips & bread, and he wants sugar - candy & goodies. Peter said he was feeling good, and he asked me how I was feeling and I realized that one of the biggest changes for me so far on this diet is that I really no longer have that afternoon lull. I always used to get so tired in the afternoon, almost falling asleep after eating lunch, but without carbs I don't feel like that.

I am sore from exercising and trying to get my body back in shape, but otherwise I feel good. I am actually enjoying the challenge of trying to find Keto friendly foods and I am excited to try some of the recipes from our new cookbook.

Day 25 –
Today was just a relaxing day because sometimes you just need that.
I actually managed to sleep in because Peter got up with the dogs.
We are still dog sitting and the sweet little visiting dog has a
tendency to get up extremely early (before 6:00am) so I have been
getting up early almost every day. Sleep is actually very important
for healthy weight. There are numerous studies that have shown a
lack of sleep is connected to weight gain.

I had my coffee and spent some time on my computer. I had some
pecans for a midmorning snack.

I made myself a big salad for lunch, with lettuce, one piece of
crumbled bacon and some feta cheese. It was yummy.

Later I did some house cleaning and Peter went shopping. I was so
excited when he brought a huge pile of produce home.

In the afternoon we went swimming and Peter noticed my ankle was
swollen, so at his insistence I put some ice on it. I think the walk to
and from the Y might have been a bit too much for my ankle. I took
today off from my workout and tomorrow I will only do the bicycle
and some weights to help give my ankle some recovery time.

For dinner we decided to try one of the new recipes out, we made
our own version of Chicken Fried rice. I really wish we could have
our own reality show it would be hilarious. We were making such a
big mess and yelling at each other and then laughing so hard. I, or
course, did not follow the recipe, but I have to say it came out so
good.

We started by cutting up the chicken into small pieces and browning
them. Peter wanted to use the griddle. We chopped up a whole bunch
of great veggies to add to our dish. After the chicken was done we
put on the broccoli, some green onions and some fresh green beans I
had cut up, next we added two beaten eggs and finally we added the
cauliflower rice and some bean sprouts. We used sesame oil and just
some onion powder, salt and pepper. It was amazing. I would
definitely make this again.

Peter and I are having fun cooking together so I am looking forward to trying more recipes.

Day 26 –
Today my goal is hydration. I want to ensure that I am fully hydrated. When you do not drink enough water, your body receives mixed signals on hunger. Dehydration causes you to believe you need to eat when you really need water. I really like that my fitbit has a tool for tracking how much water I drink. According to my fitbit I should be drinking 64 ounces of water and as you can see I have not come close to that goal. To be fair I have not always remembered to log all my water, and I have not logged other drinks like crystal light or the diet green tea that I sometimes drink.

I made myself an egg for breakfast, and really concentrated on drinking water all morning, so I had finished two full water bottles by noon, well on my way to meeting my goals. The only major downside to drinking all that water is frequently going to the bathroom.

For lunch I wanted to be brave and test out my new spiralizer. First I looked at some websites and I found this one with an easy step-by-step video (https://pinchofyum.com/8-life-changing-ways-to-use-a-spiralizer) then I prepared a cucumber to add to a salad.

I am excited to try even more recipes with my new spiralizer; maybe I can even try to do a veggie version of spaghetti.

By the early afternoon I had already finished four bottles of water! At this rate I will have no problem meeting my daily goal and hopefully even exceeding it. I want to try and meet this goal every single day this week to help make this an ongoing habit.

When Peter got home I had some of the leftover Cauliflower fried rice dish from yesterday and it was even better the second day. Peter decided he wanted to make something with chicken and mushrooms and I have no idea what he did but he just started throwing things into the pan and he came up with a bizarre concoction that he called Mexican chop suey. He said it was actually very good and he even saved some for lunch the next day.

The swelling on my ankle was down a bit, so Peter and I headed over to the Y to go workout. I skipped the treadmill and did the stationary bicycle for 20+ minutes and then I did a bunch of the weight machines. I did some arm weights and some leg machines, and I was sweating a bunch so I know I was getting both cardio and strength training. Peter said he had a great swim.

In the evening we relaxed watching some episodes of *Drunk History* and I enjoyed a glass of wine. As long as I keep it to only one glass, the 3 or 4 extra carbs are not a big deal.

It has been really great to go on this diet journey with Peter. Being able to support and encourage each other has been so helpful, and his weight loss is really starting to show. His clothes already look looser.

My weight loss is going much slower than Peter's, which I honestly expected. Men always seem to loose weight more quickly than women. I think our bodies are designed to hold on to weight – after all we are designed to give birth and feed infants, so our bodies naturally like to hang on to those stores of fat. I am going to be excited to see my total weight loss after a month. I would love to just snap my fingers or take a magic pill, but I know that weight loss is a long hard journey.

Day 27 -
I am still focusing on meeting my water goals for today. I have to really think about drinking water, so it is an effort, but I want to hit 64 ounces every single day this week.

I started my day with my usual coffee and then I made myself some scrambled eggs & cheese with a piece of bacon crumbled in. Even with just two eggs I feel satisfied, but I will admit I still do miss toast.

Now that we have been on this diet for several weeks, I am learning quite a bit more about Keto. For instance, I have been having an occasional Atkins candy snack in the evenings, but there is a big question for folks doing Keto diet whether or not they can have Atkins bars. There is a big difference between Atkins and Keto. I did some research and here is what I found out:
They're both low-carb diets, one key difference between the Keto diet and Atkins is the amount of protein you're allowed to take in. There's no cap on Atkins, while Keto limits protein to about 20 percent of your daily calories. The other big difference is that Atkins has phases, which I will explain more about below.

The Atkins approach to carbs changes over time. As the diet progresses, the carb amount allowed goes up.
In Keto you counts all carbs—not just the net—and the amount tends to be much lower long-term than that of Atkins

In the Keto diet you severely limit carbs to 50 grams or less, this diet forces your body to burn fat for energy, a process known as ketosis. Though you might feel restricted from bread and fruit, the plans emphasis on fat and protein make you feel more satisfied.

The Atkins diet has four phases. In phase one, you cut out almost all carbs, dropping your intake down to 20 grams of net carbs (carbs minus fiber = net carbs) per day, primarily from veggies. You're also required to eat protein at every meal and three servings of added fat per day. During phase two, called balancing, the daily carb allowance goes up to 50 grams of net carbs and more sources of nutrition are added. You stay in this phase until you're roughly 10 pounds away from your goal weight. Phases three and four of Atkins are all about learning to maintain your goal weight once you've reached it. Atkins sells its own line of food products, such as bars, protein drinks, and meals, that aren't entirely healthful.

Another big difference between the two is how and when both diets started.

Dr. Russell Wilder at the famous Mayo Clinic founded the ketogenic diet back in 1924. The diet was initially used for treating epilepsy. It was later realized that the Ketogenic diet was extremely effective for weight loss.

The Atkins Diet began by Dr. Robert Atkins, an American physician and cardiologist. In 1963, he discovered that reducing carbohydrate intake triggered weight loss without significant hunger, and he went on to publish his findings and diet advice in the now famous book *Dr. Atkins' Diet Revolution*.

The good news is that a **study published in** *American Family Physician* found that low-carb diets are more effective than low-fat diets at lowering levels of triglycerides and A1C and raising levels of **"good" HDL cholesterol**.
Okay so back to the original question about having Atkins treats, basically here is the consensus of my research – Low carb junk food is STILL junk food, so while those treats may help with cravings, they are not a good idea. They have very little nutritional value and they are not a good choice while on the Keto diet. I knew there were too good to be true.

Back to my boring day; I had some leftover Chicken salad for lunch. It had chicken, cheese, pecans and some raw cauliflower rice for crunch and I used avocado oil mayonnaise I found at the store. It is rich and creamy and tastes just like regular mayo but with healthy fats and no carbs.

I spent the evening hanging out with my Dad, and since I wasn't home I didn't get the chance to be more creative with my dinner so I had some tuna fish and a cucumber. I did snack on some pecans after I got home.

I am pleased to say I did meet my water goal, just barely. I really am trying to focus on taking a big drink of water a few minutes before eating anything.

For more info about the differences between Keto & Atkins you can check out these sources that I looked at.

Day 28 –
Peter and I have both been doing our low carb Keto diet for almost a full month now and I am pretty darn proud of the fact that we have stuck with it, not cheated with any of those carb-loaded goodies we crave, and we have made a real effort to include regular exercise in our lives. That really is a big accomplishment.

After my morning coffee I really wanted to give that cauliflower toast one more try and actually use parchment paper this time. I don't think I squeezed out enough liquid, but I had fun and put the batter into silly shapes with some of my cookie cutters.

They came right off the paper this time, and I had two of them. They taste okay but certainly not like real toast. I am trying to think of ways to use them, maybe with eggs, bacon and cheese on top like one of those breakfast sandwiches?

Later I had a cheese stick and did a bunch of chores around the house. No matter how often you clean and do dishes, the second you turn around there are more dishes.

I finished up some paperwork for my job, and then actually got a chance to do some reading.

When Peter came home I decided to be brave and make my own version of a Keto taco. We had some leftover cooked hamburger so I added some good 'Pico and Taco' spice to it and then proceeded to make cheese taco shells. I added the meat, some sour cream and just a small amount of salsa and they were fantastic.

Later, Peter and I headed to the YMCA and I did 45 minutes on the stationary bicycle. My ankle swelling is down but I wanted to baby it just a bit more. I will try to do some walking when I go back to the Y next time, but I will keep it at pretty low speeds to make sure that my ankle won't get too mad again.

I also managed to meet my daily water goal again. I do think drinking water is helping, but I really have to consciously think about drinking to actually meet my goal each day.

I wish I could say that my fat was just melting off but I know it's not. I also know we are making the right decisions and this will pay off, but it is going to take some time.

Day 29-
I am so grateful to be able to do this Keto journey with Peter. He makes everything more fun, and we have really enjoyed supporting and encouraging each other.

This morning I had my coffee and I was feeling hungry so I decided to have a piece of celery with some natural peanut butter on it.

It's important to get natural peanut butter to avoid any added sugars. This jar of Skippy Natural only has 6 total grams of carbs per two tablespoons, but there are 2 grams of fiber so its really only 4 net grams of carbs. Those carbs could still add up quickly so I still have to be careful how much peanut butter I have.

 After finishing some chores and phone calls for work I met Peter so he could drop his car off at the car shop and we decided to go have lunch together. Eating at a restaurant can be tricky on Keto but we were both able to make great choices.

As we walked into our favorite sports bar I noticed a sign for Cucumber Mint Vodka and I really wanted to try it. Vodka has the lowest carbs of any alcohol, so I ordered the vodka with soda and Oh My God it was amazing. I think I have found my new go-to drink. Guilt free and tastes great!

(https://www.ketelone.com/vodkas/cucumber-mint-botanical/)

I ordered a spinach salad and other than the tomatoes, which I did not eat, it was very Keto friendly and delicious. It had eggs, feta cheese and black olives. I did check to make sure the black olives were okay and yes, they are low in carbs. About 10 olives only have one net carb.

Peter had chicken wings. He is so happy that this bar doesn't serve breaded wings so these are fine to eat on Keto. We did talk about being careful eating the carrots they serve with the wings, the celery is fine but carrots actually have a lot of natural sugar; there are **6** grams of carbs per medium carrot. The blue cheese dressing is also fine on Keto so he was very happy. I had a couple wings too and they were good.

After lunch I went to get my haircut and in the evening Peter and I discussed what to have for dinner. I suggested that we try to make the zucchini noodles, so we grabbed our new Keto recipe book and decided on Zoodles with Alfredo sauce, and some Aidells sausage that we had in the freezer.

I washed the zucchini and cut off the ends, then I found the right size blade on my spiralizer and I got busy making my zoodles. The recipe said to leave them out for an hour on some parchment paper to dry out before cooking so that's what we did. Apparently parchment paper is a MUST for the Keto diet.

Peter worked on making some Alfredo sauce with butter, heavy cream and Parmesan cheese, while I prepared the zoodles. The recipe said to cook them on medium heat in a pan with some butter for 3-5 minutes until tender.

I really wasn't sure if I was going to like these zoodles but they were delicious. Seriously this meal was fabulous and I couldn't help myself I even had a little bit more for a second helping because it was so good. Peter loved it too. We saved the leftover Alfredo sauce because we saw another recipe we want to do with chicken and broccoli Alfredo.

I was so full that I didn't need or want any evening snack.

I didn't get a chance to go workout today, but as long as I work out at least every other day that's okay and it is still a big improvement from where we were a month ago. I was able to meet my daily water goal again today too so I was really happy about that. That's four days straight of at least 64 ounces of water.

Peter and I are having fun trying new recipes together, and I love that we are sticking with our carb free lifestyle.

Day 30 -
Wow – we have been on this journey for a month now. I wanted to take a moment to celebrate that commitment. I have been somewhat surprised that we have both done so well. Both Peter and I have stuck to the diet with zero cheating, which is not to say we haven't wished about and longed for all of those carb loaded goodies that we shouldn't have, but we have stuck to our diet and made healthy choices. We have also increased our exercise, and I have been regularly going to the YMCA at least every other day for the entire month. Peter has been busier with work but he has managed to go to the YMCA to swim at least 2-3 times per week.

All of that hard work has paid off. Peter has lost a total of 25 pounds so far!!! And when I checked at the YMCA today I have lost a total of 15 pounds!!!

We still have a long way to go, but that is an incredible start. And I have managed to write a daily blog post for the past 30 days too.

This morning I was busy and got totally distracted, so I skipped breakfast. I did make myself a big beautiful salad for lunch. I spiralized a cucumber and added it to some spinach, lettuce, and some pumpkin seeds.

I made time in the afternoon to go workout at the Y and did 15 minutes on the treadmill and finished with 25 minutes on the bicycle.

I am still trying to be careful with my ankle, but I set the treadmill to the 'fat burning' workout so the incline raised and lowered to increase the intensity of the workout without increasing the speed. I have enjoyed using audio books while I workout. Today I was listening to *Scrappy Little Nobody* by Anna Kendrick; she is hilarious.

For dinner I made myself some shrimp and some spinach, and Peter decided on some roasted chicken. He likes to buy the whole roasted chickens from Safeway and Costco. I did splurge on a celebratory glass of wine after dinner.

I was behind on my water consumption today. I usually finish a full bottle by noon and two or three in the afternoon. Today I had only finished one by 3:00pm, so I had to really push myself to drink all afternoon and evening. I managed to finish my full 64 ounces before bedtime. That is five straight days of meeting my goal. I have been trying to always have a water bottle with me. It's easy to drink during and after a workout, or if I go outside in the Phoenix heat, but I have to think about it at other times.

I am proud of our efforts so far, but I know that we both have a long way to go. I also know it will get harder, we will have times where we wont lose weight, we will get frustrated, but I also know that if we support each other we can do it!

Day 31 –
Today was a busy, but fun day. After my morning coffee I decided to take two pieces of the leftover cauliflower toast and heat them with some cheese on top. To be honest, they still taste nothing like toast but it was an okay breakfast. I am not sure I will make the cauliflower toast again. I have loved other cauliflower recipes but the toast just didn't work out like I had hoped.

We spent he morning cleaning the house because I was having some folks over in the afternoon to help write postcards for a local candidate that I support. Peter was so sweet and ran to the store to get snacks for us. I suggested one of those cheese trays and maybe a small veggie tray. He also came home with some Ritz crackers and a roll of summer sausage. I put out the crackers, but with 10 carbs for just 4 crackers I knew I wouldn't be having any of them. I did have a few pieces of cheese and a few slices of the sausage, both high in fat and no carbs so that was a great Keto snack.

After everyone left, Peter and I worked on dinner together. He was so excited because he had this ridiculously large tomahawk steak that he was just dying to cook. He grilled up some chicken breast for me.

We cooked some broccoli and I had a small amount of zucchini that I had cut too large for the zoodles the other night so I threw those in a pan and cooked them too. I warmed up some of the leftover Alfredo sauce and put it on the zucchini and the chicken. OMG it was amazing.

We both enjoyed our meal so much, and honestly couldn't believe this is actually a 'diet'. I think we both ate a little too much but it was soooooo good.

I looked over and saw Peter chewing on the steak bone and I started laughing, thinking how he was a perfect poster boy for the Keto diet.

After dinner we sat and watched *Avengers Infinity War, which* just came out on video today, so of course Peter had already bought it.

I topped the evening off with a glass of red wine and a very small amount of dark chocolate.

I also stayed on track with my water intake today, but I still have to think about it and remind myself to drink water. I have heard if you do a habit for three weeks straight it becomes part of your lifestyle, so I will have to keep focusing on drinking enough water. I do think the water is helping with hunger and also with my over all health, things like digestion, etc.

I didn't manage to go workout today, but I will be back at the
YMCA tomorrow. I want to keep on track because we still have lots
of weight to lose.

Day 32 –
After a month on Keto, Peter and I have become much more aware
of the sugars and carbs that are in so much of our food. I think that
is a natural side effect of this diet. I found this graphic online that
shows how much sugar is in the drinks we consume.

Just sticking to mostly water can have a significant effect on the
overall carbs and calories that you consume.

Another big change for me has been the commitment to regular
exercise. I am considering hiring a personal trainer, at least for a few
sessions so they can show me what would be the most beneficial
workout for my body and my goals. Doing a Google search can only
get you so far; sometimes you need to talk to someone with a higher
level of knowledge and expertise. I know that trainers can be
somewhat expensive, but I believe that good health is an important
investment. The key is to make the investment worth it by actually
following their advice.

Speaking of working out, Peter and I went to the YMCA to go
workout today. I did 25 minutes on the bicycle and then I did another
25 minutes on the treadmill. I have to keep my speed relatively low
because of my ankle. I am going to see my doctor to discuss what's
going on with my ankle and if I should still be having pain and
swelling two years after my injury. I know that I broke that ankle
twice and I will likely always have issues, but I just want to make
sure there isn't something else going on.

Today I started my day with my coffee and some scrambled eggs
with cheese and ham that Peter made. Then we went to workout.
Honestly I was tired, the dogs have continued to wake me up early,
so I actually took a nap. I made myself some leftovers for dinner. I
had some of the chicken that Peter grilled and I had the leftover

broccoli. I finished off the evening with one of the Nut bars and a small glass of red wine. I am fairly sure I was still well under my carb limit for the day. Peter and I have tried to keep our total daily carbs under 25 grams.

Day 33-
Since I have been writing this daily blog for over a month now, I wanted to do more than just list my daily food consumption, although I will still do that to help me stay accountable, but I also want to begin looking at some of the issues related to losing weight so today I want to talk about sleep. Not many people actually consider sleep when it comes to weight loss, yet research shows that getting adequate sleep can have a big effect on your weight and overall health. Doing your best to eat right and exercise can be sabotaged by too little sleep.

According to WebMD "Researchers found that when dieters cut back on sleep over a 14-day period, the amount of weight they lost from fat dropped by 55%, even though their calories stayed equal. ... So it's not so much that if you sleep, you'll lose weight, but that too little sleep hampers your metabolism and contributes
to weight gain."

Poor sleep has repeatedly been linked to a higher body mass index (BMI) and weight gain. This isn't great news for folks like me dealing with menopause and the obligatory night sweats. The average adult should get a minimum of eight hours of sleep, and negative effects on the body and metabolism can start when you get fewer than seven hours a night.

Some people think that staying awake longer means you will be burning more calories but that is not how the body works. Sleep is essential for a variety of your body systems. Not sleeping enough increased the likelihood of obesity by 89% in children and 55% in adults.

Even more studies show that lack of sleep can increase your appetite. Another study showed that poor sleep can decrease your resting metabolism, or the amount of calories you burn, making it even harder to lose weight.

There are many, many other studies that show the beneficial effects of adequate sleep and its relationship to weight, but I think you get the idea. If you are trying to lose weight, getting enough sleep should be just as much a priority as food choices, exercise and adequate hydration.

Here is a fun graphic I saw online with tips about getting a good night's sleep.

In terms of my diet, today was actually one of my worst days so far. Its not just that I probably exceeded my carb limit today, which I did by munching on macadamia nuts, but that I was just feeling frustrated. Today was my day to just feel discouraged. I know we have been so successful on this diet and I have lost a good amount of weight, but when I look at how much more I still have to lose it just felt overwhelming.

I think its normal to feel like that. I am so lucky that when I have those kind of days, I have an amazing support system to pick me back up. My husband and my daughter are like built in cheerleaders. Seriously, they are always happy when I say I'm heading to the YMCA. It helps a lot. I know that everyone who is trying to lose weight and improve his or her fitness level feels like this at one time or another. The key is to just stick with it. Focus on one day, one meal and one workout at a time.

I had some cheese and macadamia nuts for a morning snack. I ate a big healthy salad for lunch. I was still full hours later so I didn't cook dinner which was a mistake, because I got hungry and ate leftover summer sausage and over a cup of macadamia nuts in the evening. (They have 19 carbs for a one-cup serving). Then I broke down and had one of those unhealthy Atkins candy bars. It really wasn't a good day, but it was an important reminder to not skip meals. Hopefully I will do much better tomorrow.

As Scarlet O'Hara reminds us – "After all tomorrow is another day"

Day 34 –
What do you do after having a bad day on your diet – you get up, eat
some breakfast and go workout!

Working out really helps to elevate my mood. No matter how badly I
don't feel like going to work out, every time I do I always feel better
Usually I am a bit sore and very sweaty, but a workout always
elevates my mood. There is actually some great science behind this.
Regular exercise can relieve stress, improve memory, help you sleep
better, and boost your overall mood.

Most of us are aware of what happens to the body when we
exercise, but what exactly does exercise do to the brain?

According to a great article I read, *"If you start exercising, your
brain recognizes this as a moment of stress. As your heart
pressure increases, the brain thinks you are either fighting the
enemy or fleeing from it. To protect yourself and your brain from
stress, you release a protein called BDNF (Brain-Derived
Neurotrophic Factor). This BDNF has a protective and also
reparative element to your memory neurons and acts as a reset
switch. That's why we often feel so at ease and things are clear
after exercising and eventually happy. At the same time,
endorphins, another chemical to fight stress, is released in your
brain."*
https://www.fastcompany.com/3025957/what-happens-to-our-
brains-when-we-exercise-and-how-it-makes-us-happier

Most of us already know that endorphins are the hormones that
make you feel happy. The article was really interesting, it
explained the effect of exercise on your brain, and this image is
amazing.

After working out I came home and had some lunch. I'm all about
using up leftovers, but making them fun so I took some of the
leftover chicken breast that Peter had barbequed and warmed it in
the oven, adding some cheese on top. I also cut up a small zucchini

and spread some Parmesan on top and threw that in the oven too. It was yummy.

Later I went out to my amazing monthly book club and I decided to splurge on a cup of their Lobster Bisque, it is probably not Keto friendly but it is so yummy, creamy and spicy and full of chunks of lobster so I didn't mind cheating. I also had one glass of white wine. While I am fully committed to our diet, I also don't want the diet to completely take over my life and keep me from having fun with friends.

When I got home Peter was having a hamburger and he was so excited because my daughter found some Keto-friendly ketchup. This was so incredible because Peter was completely addicted to ketchup. Ketchup is probably the one thing he missed the most while on this diet, he nearly cried when she gave it to him

He said it tastes good, and with only one carb per serving he is a very happy man.

One final positive note for today – I met my water goal once again. I may not be perfectly doing Keto, but I am working toward my long-term health goals.

Day 35-
My weight loss is stuck right now, so I am trying to give it a kick-start by increasing my exercise when I can. Today, after my morning coffee and some scrambled eggs, I finished a few chores and headed to the YMCA.

I was a little concerned about my ankle swelling after walking so much yesterday, so I started with the bicycle for 30 minutes and then I finished off with 20 minutes on the treadmill.

I tried the elliptical, but the ones at our YMCA are just not comfortable for me. I feel very unstable on it. Part of the reason I am unstable is due to a torn ACL ligament from the same injury where I broke my ankle the second time. What can I say I am an over achiever. It doesn't really present any major problems not having the ACL but I do have less stability than most folks. Add my extra weight and the fact that I am over 50 and you get far less balance and stability.

Finding the right exercise that you enjoy is important. My hubby loves to swim, so doing some laps is great for him. He challenges himself with how far he will swim for each workout. I like to swim casually, but I'm not a very strong swimmer so doing laps would not be my choice. I do have a friend who wants me to come to Zumba with her, so I may have to give that a try. I have heard from lots of folks how much fun they have with Zumba. Once the weather begins to cool just a bit I can go back to walking outside, and hopefully soon I will feel ready to get back into hiking too.

After I got home from the YMCA, I made myself a lovely piece of fish with lemon-butter sauce and some asparagus. It was delicious.

In the afternoon Peter got home early so we spent some time in our pool, it was a little cloudy so it was perfect.

I had lots of fun in the evening going to one of those Paint & Sip events with some friends. I decided to drink some vodka as a good low carb choice, and I split a veggie and hummus tray with a friend, she ate the hummus & pita and I got to munch on the celery and cucumbers with some ranch dressing. It does take some work, but it is possible to make healthy Keto choices even when eating out.

I was a little hungry when I got home so I snacked on a few pieces of cheese and a handful of pecans.

Day 36 –
Despite our best-laid plans, sometimes life just happens. Today was one of those interesting days. I had every intention of going to work out in the morning, but instead my plans changed and I spent the afternoon hanging out with my dad. He is 89 years old and he

lives with my amazing brother and sister-in-law. Today my sister-in-law was out of town caring for her own dad, so when my brother called I came over to be with my dad.

I stopped at the store on the way, because I wanted to make sure I had something Keto friendly to eat. I really struggled to find something that sounded appetizing and was also a good source of the fat and protein I needed without the carbs. I actually settled on a small dish of a Mediterranean salad of olives and feta cheese in an olive oil dressing. It worked great, and I wasn't hungry at all for the rest of the afternoon.

After my brother got home from work I headed home. Peter had waited for me to get home before he ate so we had fun cooking together. I made myself some zoodles, and had them with some shrimp and Alfredo sauce.

Peter made himself a steak with a big pile of sautéed mushrooms and some of the zoodles.

It was so good, and we really had fun cooking together. One of the things that work really well for us is to not necessarily worry about eating the same thing. Peter has always liked steak much more than I ever will. I don't mind an occasional filet, but I would honestly always prefer a good piece of fish or other seafood any day. The ability to enjoy our time cooking together doesn't mean we always have to eat the same things.

While I did manage to meet my water goal, I didn't get a chance to go workout today. I do feel like we are settling in to a comfortable routine with our diet and exercise. Hopefully that will translate into continued weight loss and improved health.

Day 37 –
It feels strange to be writing day 37, that means Peter and I have been sticking with this diet for 37 days so far, and I have actually been writing a daily blog post about it for 37 days. That's the good news; the not great news for me anyway is that I have

completely stopped losing weight, even with trying to increase my exercise. When I checked my weight I was actually up 2 pounds. I am still down a total of 11 pounds but I have so much more to go. I think this forces me to look at what I am eating, and how much I am eating and make some adjustments.

Lazy Keto may have only gotten me so far, and this is very hard for me because I am definitely not a 'count calories and measure my food' kind of person. I will need to be much more aware of smaller portions. There is so much information out there about Keto, and it can get a little overwhelming, but I know there are folks who are having great results so I think it is worth a little effort.

I am not going to lie; being completely stuck in my weight loss, even though I have not cheated at all is super frustrating. I was pretty grumpy, but luckily with Peter's help and support I was able to change my attitude.

I started my day at the YMCA, doing the stationary bicycle for twenty minutes.

Then I did thirty minutes on the treadmill. I am continuing to keep it at a lower speed but increasing my incline for more intensity. I did ask about having someone help me with a workout routine, but I have not gotten that scheduled yet.

Peter and I went out to lunch and I had a Cobb salad. I asked them to make it without tomatoes and everything else, egg, bacon, chicken, olives and lettuce was Keto friendly.

Peter could tell I needed some cheering up so we had a fun date night at Zzeeks and we enjoyed trying their broccoli & cheese crust. It was good, but I like the Cauliflower crust just a bit better. https://zzeeks.com/broccoli-cheddar-crust/ It has 26 grams of carbs for two slices of pizza so that is still on the high side but we both decided that it was okay to take a break once in awhile and today I really needed a break. In fact some dieting experts believe that a cheat meal high in calories and carbohydrates can actually assist jumpstarting your metabolism and regulating these hormones.

I also found this amazing Low carb ice cream. Peter had some in the evening. I didn't have any, but I did taste Peter's and it was really good.

At only 12 grams of carbs per serving this is a really awesome way to treat ourselves once in awhile and still stay on our diet.
I am working on an attitude adjustment and trying to think more about long-term health rather than just about short-term weight loss. It is hard to not compare myself to Peter. The weight just seems to be falling off him. My goal this week is to continue to make sure I am getting my necessary water, and to focus on decreasing my portion sizes. Hopefully that, along with exercise, will help me start to lose again.

Day 38 –
I woke up today with a much better attitude. It never helps anything to beat yourself up, especially over things you really can't control. This morning I had some coffee and Peter made some scrambled eggs with ham. I ate a few bites, but I really wasn't feeling hungry so I put the rest of my portion in some Tupperware for tomorrow. I am trying to be more aware of portion sizes and of only eating when I feel hungry.

I got busy doing a writing project all morning and before I knew it, it was late afternoon. After helping Peter with a household project, we both didn't feel like cooking so we went to our favorite local sports bar. Peter had some wings. He loves that he can have the wings at his favorite place because there is no breading on their wings, so they are Keto friendly. I chose cheddar crusted chicken and asked for two vegetables instead of the potatoes or rice that usually comes with the meal, so I got broccoli and green beans.

We were enjoying talking and took our time eating, and after I finished the broccoli and about half of the chicken, I put my fork down and brought the remainder home for leftovers.

I didn't get a chance to go workout but I still feel really good about my food choices today. I know that as life gets busier this fall I will struggle to find time to workout as often, but if I can manage at least 3-4 days a week that will still be okay. I can also do small things every day, like take the stairs instead of an elevator or park further away from the front door when I go places. The important part is making an effort at moving more.

Day 39 –
Today was busier than usual; I had to rush out early to stop by work before spending the day with my Dad. I managed to grab a cup of coffee and I warmed the scrambled eggs from yesterday, but I wasn't too hungry so I only had a few bites and then I shared the rest with my very appreciative dog.

Spending time with my Dad is always great, but not being at home makes it harder to stay on my routine. While dad had his lunch I grabbed a cheese stick and a few pieces of turkey. I also had a handful of Crisps that I brought with me. One of the helpful things I have been doing is trying to remember to pack healthy Keto snacks to take with me if I leave home. I also snacked on some pecans in the afternoon when I got hungry.

After I got home I cooked a piece of salmon and some cauliflower rice, and I also snacked on a few more Crisps and pecans in the evening.

I am trying to balance focusing on smaller portion sizes with feeling hungry, so I am working on finding the perfect amount that is just enough, not too much or too little.

One of the things that many overweight people struggle with is portion size. It is so difficult to stop eating - especially when something tastes really good. I remember my Mom once telling me

she didn't have an 'enough' button so she would always just keep
eating. I think we all do have an 'enough' button but some of us
just stop listening to it. If you watch most small children, they will
eat large amounts of food one day, and barely anything another
day. When adults offer healthy choices and don't try to force their
eating, small children do an incredible job of regulating their diet.
Somewhere along the line we lose that ability.

That's my goal this week, along with exercise and water; I am
going to work on re-discovering my 'enough' button.

Day 40 –
Wow, we made it forty days so far. We didn't survive a flood like
Noah, but we have resisted temptation for the most part and have
stuck with our diet.

I had a conversation with Peter and my daughter and I have
decided to commit to 100 days of Keto. For me, saying I will stick
with this for a year or indefinitely is just too big and too long and I
will lose hope. 100 days is a really long time, and it should help
make a big difference in my weight loss journey, but I just can't
see avoiding all carbs indefinitely. Since we have already
completed 40 days that only leaves 60 days left, or two full months
and that seems reasonable to me. I can do that!

This does not mean that after 100 days I will open 2 bags of potato
chips and start pigging out, it just means that I will include more
variety into my diet, including more fruits and veggies that we are
completely avoiding right now, as well as dairy and some whole
grains. I still have a lot to lose, so even with two more months of
Keto I won't be at my goal weight.

Speaking of weight, with my very close attention to portion sizes I
am starting to slowly creep back down on the scale. Portion size is
something I will have to pay attention to for the rest of my life.
Getting older, especially for women after menopause, causes our
body's metabolism to slow down. Even with exercise, we simply

do not burn the same amount of calories as we did when we were younger.

According to WebMD, it is our lack of estrogen that is the culprit.

> ***The impact of estrogen.*** *In animal studies, estrogen appears to help control body weight. With lower estrogen levels, lab animals tend to eat more and be less physically active. Reduced estrogen may also lower metabolic rate, the rate at which the body converts stored energy into working energy. It's possible the same thing happens with women when estrogen levels drop after menopause. Some evidence suggests that estrogen hormone therapy increases a woman's resting metabolic rate. This might help slow weight gain. Lack of estrogen may also cause the body to use starches and blood sugar less effectively, which would increase fat storage and make it harder to lose weight.*
> https://www.webmd.com/menopause/guide/menopause-weight-gain-and-exercise-tips#1

In addition, you lose muscle mass as you get older, which lowers your resting metabolism. Women are really fighting a much harder battle. That is why Peter is able to lose so much more than I am. I try really hard not to compare myself to Peter, and I am genuinely happy about his fantastic weight loss so far.

I spent the day with my dad again, so my normal routine was off, but I still kept my portions small. After my morning coffee I made myself two eggs. Then I went over to my brother's house for the day. While I was there I snacked on some pecans and I had one of those yummy nut rolls in the afternoon. It really did the trick and filled me up. After I got home I finished off the leftover chicken and green beans from the other night, and a small amount of leftover salmon from the night before. Later I had a small handful of Crisps while watching TV. Sometimes I really like to have something crunchy and those Crisps have been perfect.

The only bummer about today was that I just did not have time to go workout, but that's okay. I will do my best to get back on track and head over to the YMCA first thing tomorrow morning.

I am feeling much more positive this week, and I hope the scale will reflect my renewed enthusiasm.

Day 41-
After my morning coffee I did some work and then grabbed a quick cheese stick for protein and headed to the YMCA. I did 20 minutes on the stationary bicycle, but my headphones stopped working so I took this as a sign to skip the treadmill and go use the weight machines. I really need the distraction of music or an audio book when I use the treadmill.

I was motivated to work on building muscle mass after my research yesterday on metabolism and older women. I know building muscle is important for health and long lasting weight loss so I did eight arm machines and four leg machines and I certainly worked up a sweat.

When I got home I made myself some tuna for lunch. I added some cauliflower rice for crunch.

Later I jumped in the shower and headed out to work for the afternoon. I was hungry when I got home so I used my spiralizer and made some zoodles, which I had with some leftover chicken and alfredo sauce. It was so yummy, but I was careful to only serve myself half of what I made and save the second half for tomorrow. I am really focusing on keeping a reasonable portion size, so I felt proud that even though it tasted great, I did not let myself overeat.

I am still keeping a food journal each day. It helps me to keep track of my diet for the blog as well as keeping me accountable for what I eat. When I see it written down it does make a difference. I think sometimes its easy to lie to ourselves and say, "I didn't eat that much" but when you see it in black and white it really makes a difference. I also track my exercise.

Day 42 –

Another busy day, which actually helped keep me on track. I started out the day with my usual cup of coffee and then after some work, including a boring conference call for work. Right after the conference call I ran over to the YMCA because at that point I really needed to move.

Since I focused on weights yesterday, today I just did the treadmill, but I wound up walking for 50 minutes.

I was really pleased when I stepped on the scale and I am back on track with weight loss. This was really motivating to see.

Portion control really is everything, so I decided to do a little research about portion sizes. I found this photo comparing plate sizes, no wonder Americans are overweight. We simply eat more food.

I found a great blog post discussing ways to reduce portion sizes. (https://skinnyms.com/6-easy-ways-to-reduce-portion-sizes/)

Here are the six tips they shared
1. Use a Smaller Plate – this one is obvious it makes your amount of food look like more; it's a mental trick to help you not eat as much.
2. Leave a Few Bites Behind – this one is much harder for those of us who were taught to clean our plates, but it is still a good goal.
3. Share – this one was mostly referring to restaurants where the portions are notoriously large, so share with someone. I used to do that sometimes with my daughters when going out to eat.
4. Up the Greens – this one is self-explanatory; veggies are always a better choice.
5. Pre-Portion Snacks – this actually does help, don't bring over a whole package of something, just put a small amount in a cup, that way you have to consciously choose to eat more.
6. Use Your Knife – here they were talking about cutting up your portions so you take more time eating, and it feels like more because there are more pieces.

I think these are all good suggestions. Overall the main point is to be mindful of your portions when eating and try to focus on how much you are eating.

After working out I had the leftover zoodles with chicken and Parmesan that I had saved from the night before. It was perfect and filled me up.

I went to volunteer in the evening and I was so happy that they had some peanuts in their snack pile this time. I had about a half cup of peanuts and that really seemed to work well. I wasn't really hungry when I got home and it was already after 8:00pm so I decided to just skip dinner.

After being on the diet for 42 days now, some of these habits are becoming easier – it just feels natural to always have my water bottle with me, or to count the number of carbs in something when I grocery shop. I am hoping that these habits will just be part of my life after my 100 days commitment.

Day 43 –
I really wanted to get over to the YMCA today, but I just ran out of time. With work and chores and other commitments I just couldn't get there, but its okay – I will definitely make time to go tomorrow.

I had a busy morning so I just grabbed some coffee and ran out of the house, I was gone until after noon so when I got home I made myself some cauliflower rice and leftover chicken. It was just enough to fill me up.

I juggled several more commitment and didn't get home until after seven at night. Peter was barbequing a steak for himself so I had him throw on a bratwurst for me and we decided to try and grill some asparagus. I tossed them in some olive oil and a few spices and threw them on the grill. They were so good.

I started using a smaller size lunch plate. I want to follow my own advice. I also carefully cut up the bratwurst into small bite size pieces and honestly it did work. I felt full when I finished. Every little trick to reduce portions is a good thing right now.

Peter said he feels like he is stuck in his weight loss right now so he is going to work on reducing his portion sizes too and I am going to encourage him to come workout with me more. It is hard because I have been busy the past few evenings and that is when Peter can go workout. He always seems more motivated when we go together. I am going to have to be careful to say no to some of my commitments to protect that evening time for Peter and I to workout together. Even though he goes and swims and I use the machines – just driving over there together is motivating for both of us.

Last year we worked hard at making sure our finances were in order, and we have both decided that this year's goal is our health and fitness so I want to make sure that working towards good health is our priority right now. Like a lot of women I have a hard time saying no to things, but I will try.

Making time for exercise and continuing to work on eating right is our goal and our commitment to each other.

Day 44 –
So today I got completely distracted with work, I had so much going on and I simply ran out of time to eat. I realized it was 1:30 and I had not eaten at all. I was actually starting to not feel well and unfortunately I had forgotten to plan ahead and have my healthy snacks with me.

Apparently I had unintentionally done intermittent fasting. Many Keto experts recommend at least some fasting for individuals on the Keto diet, primarily to help achieve ketosis. Some experts believe that intermittent fasting may drive blood-sugar levels down, which can promote or enhance ketosis.

After reading several articles about fasting on the Keto diet, here is what I learned: It's not necessary to do intermittent fasting on the Keto diet but it may help, especially for folks who have reached a plateau with their weight loss. Doing intermittent fasting on the Keto diet *can* speed up fat burn and weight loss.

If you have ever had a day where you ate dinner before 8 p.m. but didn't eat or drink anything with calories until noon the next day? Then you've intermittently fasted. If you had to do blood work that required fasting or had to fast before a medical procedure, then you have done intermittent fasting.

All of the articles were very clear that if you have diabetes and use insulin, or are following a Keto diet for medical reasons like epilepsy, you definitely shouldn't practice intermittent fasting (or even do Keto, for that matter) without talking to a nutritionist who specializes in the diet first.

It can be overwhelming because there is so much information out there, but it is especially important to look for reliable sources, no just some self-proclaimed expert.

So after unintentionally fasting, I came home and had a leftover bratwurst and a cheese stick. Then Peter got home and we both went to the YMCA.

I had a great workout; I started with 15 minutes on the stationary bicycle for a warm up. Then I did a circuit of the weight machines. Finally I finished off with 10 minutes on the treadmill waiting for Peter to finish.

After we got home I jumped in the pool to cool off and then made myself some shrimp and cauliflower rice for dinner. I am still using smaller plates and focusing on smaller portion sizes.

Day 45 –

I made a mistake last night and had a bottle of sugar free green tea in the evening and I had a lot of trouble falling asleep. I was feeling sluggish all day. I had my usual morning coffee and decided to make myself a fried egg for breakfast.

In addition to feeling tired, I had a huge to-do list today, including teaching a class, so I stayed busy all morning. When I returned home in the afternoon I ate some of the leftover shrimp and cauliflower rice and then I took a nap. I am not usually inclined to take naps, but sometimes you have to listen to your body signals. My body was clearly telling me I needed some time to rest and recuperate. Sleep is incredibly restorative.

I still felt a little sluggish when I woke up. Peter had barbecued a whole chicken, and made more cauliflower rice. I helped and made some of the Parmesan zucchini chips.

Despite my nap I went to bed early, my body was clearly trying to tell me I had been too busy the past few days and that I needed to slow down a bit. Although I didn't get a chance to make it to the YMCA, my fitbit assured me I had done plenty of walking all day long.

I know that I am often guilty of overscheduling myself. It is hard to say no, or even give myself permission to have a simple day of rest, but we all need those days sometimes.

I am so proud of Peter, even though he was tired and sore from his swim yesterday, he went to the YMCA while I was working and he swam again. He told me it was hard at first but after a few laps it felt really good. He and I are planning to go to the YMCA again tomorrow.

Supporting and encouraging each other on this diet journey has been so great. I know I would not have been as successful on this diet without his help. It sounds strange to say, but doing this together has actually been fun. We have both worked really hard to be a positive role model for each other, and we have been careful not to nag or scold the other for their choices. Staying positive is the key. Offering positive feedback when we each make good choices is what really works. I am so lucky to have such a great guy.

Day 46 –
I slept in this morning and when I woke up Peter made me breakfast. Along with my coffee I had a delicious bacon and cheese omelet. Of course Peter put a huge pile of bacon on my plate. He is very heavy-handed when he does portions, but I only ate 2 pieces and saved the rest for other uses this week, like adding it to salad.

After breakfast we relaxed for a bit and then headed over to the YMCA. I did 40 minutes on the treadmill. Tomorrow I will do weight machines again. Peter has gone swimming for three days straight, swimming over 1000 meters each day. He is really motivated and says the swimming is coming easier now.

Peter said people have been noticing his weight loss. Not so much yet for me, but of course I have not lost as much weight as he has. We were talking about it and I explained that my body simply does not burn as many calories as his. I know I am not alone, but it doesn't make it any less frustrating. If I ate the same portions as Peter I would immediately start gaining weight, even though he is losing weight. It doesn't seem fair, but it is reality.

After we finished our workout we headed over to Costco for some shopping. It was a struggle going down aisles with all those yummy but forbidden carbs. It was interesting how carefully both of us checked each package for the number of carbs.

We had not eaten lunch so we were tempted by all of the samples offered, and we did indulge on some of the samples. I am sure we had a few more carbs then we should have, but we did share our small sample cups so it was fewer carbs then taking a whole sample. We tried some shrimp pesto pasta salad and I had one shrimp and one noodle, Peter actually had 3 small noodles. We tried some

Hawaiian chicken that I know had some sugar in the sauce, but I only ate one bite and Peter tried a small bite but he didn't like it. We were more than happy to try several of the Aidelles sausage samples because those were fairly safe, and Peter wound up buying some of those. I did eat one healthy tortilla chip.

There was something fun about having a small amount of forbidden foods. After 45 days of an extremely low carb diet, we both decided a small sample or two would not be the biggest crime. It is important to live in balance and we did skip several samples that we knew would not be a good idea including the bread and waffles. We left Costco with a cart full of healthy food choices.

After returning home and putting away the groceries we jumped into the pool for a swim, and then Peter started up the barbeque for dinner. He mad himself a cube steak with some grilled onion, I had a piece of salmon and I made a big tray of oven roasted broccoli and cauliflower. It came out great. I did snack on a handful of pecans after dinner.

I have been a bit lax in my water consumption the past couple days so I will have to really focus on that again this week. I know that drinking enough water will continue to help in my weight loss.

Day 47 –
I began my day with coffee and worked on my computer for a few hours. When I finally got hungry I warmed up some of the leftover Parmesan zucchini chips from the other night along with a piece of salmon. After finishing I ate a handful of Crisps to satisfy that need for a crunchy treat.

Today was just one of those busy kind of days where you work for hours and don't feel like you got anything done. In the afternoon I headed over to the YMCA. I was a bit frustrated because I tried to use my Bluetooth headphones but as soon as I put them on I heard the voice said "battery low". Even without an audiobook, I stayed on the stationary bicycle for about 35 minutes.

I decided to go and step on the scale and I am excited to announce that I have lost a total of 18 pounds since starting the diet. All of my effort at smaller portions and being consistent with exercise is starting to pay off. I am hoping to reach a total of 20 pounds by the end of the month.

It is important to take some time to celebrate victories and losing eighteen pounds is a big deal. I found this silly meme that shows 18 pounds is the same as six steam irons.

After getting home from working out, I made myself a piece of fish with lemon and butter sauce and some asparagus with some Parmesan sprinkled on top. It was really good. I am still using smaller plates and really focusing on the amount that I eat.

I did have a nut bar in the evening while we watched TV. I was really craving something sweet, and the nut bar is perfect for that. I knew I had not gone over my carb limit for the day so I decided it was okay to have one.

Sometimes it feels like we have been on this diet forever, but I can see that it is working so I just have to keep on making good healthy choices.

Day 48 –
I grabbed some coffee and packed a small container of pecans for work this morning. I am only working a half-day so the pecans should be enough to get me through until lunch.

When I got home I made myself a salad with some cucumber, and then I decided to try a new Keto recipe.

I was really excited when we went to Costco a few days ago because they had almond flour, which is essentially just ground up almonds, but it makes a good flour substitute in Keto recipes.

We also got some cacao powder, again basically just unsweetened chocolate that is used in many keto recipes.

I felt like these would give us more variety in our options of what to cook.

The one thing I miss the most is the crunch of crackers or chips so I decided to make some low carb cheese crackers (see recipe below).

I used one cup of Parmesan and one cup of cheddar for my cheese choices. The recipe was fairly simple to follow.

Low Carb Cheese Crackers Recipe

- 2 Cups Cheese of your choice (I used a Parmesan-Romano mix along with some Swiss and cheddar)
- 1 cup **Almond Flour**
- 2 oz. Cream Cheese
- 1 egg
- 1/2 teaspoon sea salt
- 1 teaspoon Rosemary (or a seasoning of your choice such as basil, chives, garlic, dill weed, spicy chili, thyme, oregano etc.,)

1. Mix all the cheeses (including the cream cheese) along with the **almond flour in a microwave safe bowl and cook it for exactly one** minute. (UPDATE: There are some people that prefer not to use a microwave and I certainly understand that. You can heat these ingredients up on the stovetop too. You are going to heat them up just enough for the cheese to my melted enough for you to roll out the dough.
I would continue stirring it while heating it up on the stovetop.)
2. Immediately stir the ingredients until the almond flour and cheeses have combined fully. You want the cheese to be partially melted (see photo)
3. Allow this to cool for a few minutes because if you put the egg in these ingredients too soon it will cook the egg.
4. Now add the egg, sea salt, and seasoning of your choice. I decided to cut up some fresh rosemary I had on hand. You

want to add about a teaspoon of your favorite seasoning unless it's a spicy mix. I would add only about a 1/2 teaspoon for spicy seasonings.

5. Mix it together until all the ingredients are fully combined. If you cheese has gotten too hard or it's too hard to mix, you can microwave your cheese for another 20 seconds to get it soft again.

6. Now you will place the ball of dough on a large sheet of **parchment paper. Then place another sheet of parchment paper of** equal size on top of the ball of dough.

7. You can use your hands or a rolling pin to spread the dough out into a thin layer. It spread so easily that I used my hands to have more control and keep the dough inside the square piece of parchment paper. Make sure the parchment paper is the same size as your baking sheet.

8. Next, use a pizza cutter to cut the crackers into small squares as seen in the photos.

9. Bake these crackers on each side at 450 degrees for about 5 or 6 minutes on each side. If the crackers are thin, you will cook them about 5 minutes on each side but if the dough is thick, it may take 7 to 9 minutes to get the crispy cracker texture you are looking for. When you keep the dough on the parchment paper it's really easy to flip it over while it's hot after cooking it on the first side. I ended up using the pizza cutter again to define the lines on the flip side too. Feel free to leave the crackers in the oven longer (but watch them closely) if you love a very crispy texture. The crispier the better for me!

10. Allow the crackers to cool for about 5 minutes and they are ready to eat!

I thought they came out great, especially the slightly burnt ones on the edge. I think my dough was a bit too thick because some of the ones in the middle were not quite crispy, but they tasted great.

It was really fun to try a new recipe.

Peter didn't get home until later – so I headed over to the YMCA without him. I did 40 minutes on the treadmill.   As long as I keep my speed at about 2.5 my ankle seems to do okay, but I do wonder if I will ever be able to do the running and hiking I used to do. I am hoping that once I lose a bunch of this extra weight I might be able to do more.

I jumped in the pool when I got home and then had some fun with dinner. I took some leftover chicken and cut it up into small pieces. I threw the chicken in a pan with a bunch of Penzies chicken taco spice and then added a small can of green chili enchilada sauce. As it got warm I added just a bit of cream cheese and some sour cream. The sauce was so rich and creamy. Next I made the cheese enchilada shells in the over (4 small circles of cheddar cheese on parchment paper, cooked at 350 degrees for seven minutes). I am getting pretty good at rolling the cheese shells and it was delicious. I made some for Peter when he got home too. I have to admit it was so good I did not limit my portions tonight.

I looked at a calendar today, and our 100 days will end in October. That's great because I have travel plans to go on an amazing trip in October. My friend and I are going to Thailand. That was actually a big factor in wanting to do this diet. I wanted to lose weight and get in shape before our trip.

We have almost finished halfway to our 100 days. I don't plan to simply return to our old lifestyle after 100 days, we will continue to watch our carbs, avoid processed foods – especially sugar and white flour, and we will continue to make healthy choices with exercise, portion sizes and everything else we have learned from doing this diet.

Day 49 -
I am excited that we are almost halfway through our 100 days and we are still going strong, in fact I think we are getting better at staying Keto.

I really wanted to take Lexi out for a walk this morning, it looked like it was cloudy so I was hopeful, but when I went outside the sidewalk was already hot to the touch. I guess taking walks out side will have to wait a few more weeks before it finally cools down enough. Instead, after my morning coffee I went over the YMCA and jumped on the stationary bike.

I did only about 30 minutes but I did not stay and do the weight machines, because I really had a bunch of work to finish today.

I did decide to check my weight and I was really happy to see I am down another pound.

I know it's not just about weight loss, but losing weight is a tangible way to see the positive results of the diet so far.

When I got home I made myself a big salad, with some feta cheese and some pumpkin seeds for crunch.

Later I made myself a couple more of the cheese enchiladas with the leftovers from yesterday. It was great. I did also snack on some of the Keto cheese crackers I had made. The were not as crunchy as I hoped, and I am not sure if putting them in the fridge was part of the reason why, but since they are made of cheese I thought keeping them in the fridge was a good idea.

I spent some time looking for fun Keto recipes online and I noticed someone posted about a documentary on Netflix called *The Magic Pill*. I asked Peter if he was interested and we watched it. It was all about several people who were on the Keto diet and we both enjoyed watching it. I know Keto goes against some conventional nutrition advice, but I can't argue with the results.

Day 50 -
It just so happens that day 50, exactly halfway through my personal challenge of 100 days on Keto, is also my birthday. I have decided to allow myself a cheat day, but despite that fact I had to work all day so I packed myself a healthy lunch with a salad and some healthy Keto snacks including a small container of pecans and another small container of Crisps.

At work I saw someone had a big bag of Candy. Gosh it's not even September yet and already the Halloween candy is everywhere. I decided to take a look at the number of carbs and in one small bite-sized candy is 22-32 carbs, depending on the type of candy. YIKES! So eating any of these candies would put me over my daily carb limit. This diet really has made me more aware of the amount of carbs in food. There is no question that all of these processed and sugary foods are the cause of not only obesity, but also the cause of so many other related health problems including diabetes, hypertension and so much more.

I started my day by grabbing some coffee and munching on a cheese stick. Lunch was a salad with feta and pumpkin seeds again, and I had some Crisps. I did snack on a few pecans in the afternoon.

After work I met a friend for a birthday happy Hour and this is where I decided to splurge just a bit. I ordered myself a Pear Blossom Martini. My friend and I shared a plate of cauliflower nachos and it was really good. It actually filled me up and that's all I had. It was funny actually, because I had given myself permission to cheat, but I really didn't feel like it. I am so committed to this goal that I just don't want to eat junk right now. We had so much fun making plans for our upcoming trip to Thailand, and I was so excited about everything we would do and see there – even more reason to lose weight and get in good shape.

Peter had made himself some ribs for dinner and he was so proud of them that when I got home I tried one of the ribs and they were good. I did have a few small pieces of dark chocolate as a birthday treat in the evening. I still do crave something sweet in the evening, but just one or two small pieces is usually enough to satisfy my cravings.

Day 51 –
I am excited to be starting the second half of this Keto journey.

I was running late this morning so I had to grab a cup of coffee and rush out of the house, but I did manage to quickly grab several healthy Keto snacks for my lunch. I had two cheese sticks, some of those Keto cheese crackers that I made, a small container of pecans and some Crisps. I am not sure if my meal was very balanced, but it was plenty of food to get me through the day.

After work Peter took me out for a special birthday dinner and we both had a BIG cheat night.

My main cheat was several of these incredibly delicious Pineapple Martini's. They were absolutely amazing and I am fairly certain that just having one was over my daily limit of carbs and I wound up having THREE of them, but they were so good.

We both ordered surf and turf entrees and mine was fabulous. My meal was actually pretty good in terms of Keto, but I ate way more than I have been eating lately because it was just so delicious. I did wind up bringing home most of the sirloin and green beans. Peter did have Parmesan mashed-potatoes with his meal and yes I did have to try a forkful, they were amazing.

Our biggest cheat of the night was a piece of crème brulee cheesecake that we shared as my birthday treat. I don't even want to guess how many carbs were in it, but I enjoyed eating every single carb in it.

I know that was a really big splurge, but it is important to not let any diet take over your whole life. Sometimes it is okay to throw caution to the wind and just enjoy yourself, especially on a special occasion. The big challenge is making sure that you don't do this too often.

We both felt a little guilty for not sticking with our Keto plan, so I did a bit of research and I found out this is not too big of a setback. According to ruled.me.com "In general, you will probably be back in ketosis within the next **24 to 48 hours** if one or more of the following applies to you: You were in ketosis for around a month or longer before cheating on the diet. You are doing an extended intermittent fast (>**16 hours**) beginning after your last cheat meal."

Tomorrow we will both be back on track with our diet.

Day 52 –
After such a big splurge last night I have to admit that this morning
my tummy was unhappy. I did eat one friend egg for breakfast to
settle my stomach, but it didn't really work. I felt a bit yucky all
morning – the price I had to pay for our cheat meal.

I did finally start to feel a little better in the afternoon so I heated up
my leftover green beans and filet. I did not make it over to the
YMCA today, but I am planning to go tomorrow.

Peter really wanted to try some of those 'fat bomb' recipes that I had
mentioned to him. Although something called a 'fat bomb' sounds
really strange, fat bombs are used by lots of folks on the Keto diet to
ensure they are eating an adequate amount of fat.

According to ruledme.com, "Fat bombs are a delicious combination
of ketogenic ingredients that you can have as a snack, dessert, or
meal replacement." I have seen a lot about them on Keto Facebook
groups, but we haven't tried any yet so this will be something new.
Not everyone on Keto has to or needs to eat fat bombs, but if you are
concerned about not having enough fat in your diet these are a good
ay to jump your fat consumption up quickly.

Peter and Danielle helped and we had a fun family day in the kitchen
with our new food processor.

Peter started by making a Keto Guacamole/Bacon fat bomb. Peter is
happy to make anything that involves bacon.
Here is the link for that recipe:
https://ketodietapp.com/Blog/lchf/Bacon-Guacamole-Fat-Bombs

Next we made Pecan Pie fat bombs. I happen to absolutely love
Pecan pie so I was excited to try these and luckily my adorable
healthy vegan daughter had all the ingredients we needed. We all
had fun playing with the new food processor.

According to the recipe, " they're gluten-free, grain-free, paleo,

vegan, Whole30-approved, AND Keto if you leave out the date. They're loaded with healthy fats, so just one ball will help keep you full for a while." We did change the recipe slightly; we subtracted from recipe: shredded coconut & coconut butter.
We also exchanged peanut butter for the pecan butter and artificial sugar for the date. It is important to not over-process the pecans or you will wind up with nut butter. These tasted good, but they had a little but of a gritty feel to them.

Here is the link for that recipe:
https://www.bakerita.com/pecan-pie-fat-bombs/

Next we made some ridiculously rich chocolate peanut butter balls. We accidently added all the ingredients together at first in the food processor instead of sprinkling the chocolate over the top, but I think they still came out nicely. I left them in the freezer for almost a half hour but they were still a bit loose to roll into balls. I did like the one I tasted. It was very rich and chocolaty, but not very sweet.
Here is the link for that recipe:
https://www.delish.com/cooking/recipe-ideas/recipes/a58139/keto-fat-bombs-recipe/

I didn't try one of the Bacon Guacamole ones yet – two fat bombs in one day were more than enough. It was fun to make these and hopefully they will help us ensure adequate fat intake.

Day 53 –
We were both feeling better today, so it's time to return to the good eating habits that were getting such good results.

I started my day with my coffee as usual and I decided to snack on one of the Pecan Pie fat bombs that we made yesterday to help jump-start my fat for the day.

I helped with some chores and worked on my blog and for lunch I decided to have some egg salad. I also snacked on a handful of Crisps with that.

In the evening Peter made himself a wonderful dish with chicken, mushrooms he had sautéed and some cauliflower rice. I didn't have any because I really don't like mushroom so I chose to make myself some cauliflower rice and one of the Aidelle's sausages we got at Costco last week. I chopped the sausage and it really helped to give the cauliflower rice a nice flavor.

I had one of the yummy chocolate fat bombs as my 'dessert' while we were watching TV and relaxing in the evening.

I did not make it over to the YMCA; I was still not quite feeling great. I think both Peter and I had a small resurgence of our 'Keto Flu' after my special birthday dinner. I do think it is okay to have an indulgence once in awhile, but it is hard on Keto because it take a few days to recover and get back to our new normal.

We still have a long way to go in order to reach our goals, but we are getting there.

Day 54 –
My morning started with an early doctor's appointment for my annual physical and I was so pleased to be able to tell my doctor that I have lost at least 15 pounds so far in the past two months. My weight does fluctuate from day to day and I know that our splurge for my birthday set me back a pound or two, but I could tell my doctor was impressed when I shared what I had been doing. I will be getting some blood work tomorrow and I will be very interested to see if there are any challenges related to our Keto diet, but I don't think there will be. I really do feel good overall and I know I am getting in shape.

When I got home I made myself a simple salad with some lettuce and then I got really busy with work for the rest of the afternoon.

When Peter got home we both started working on dinner. Peter made himself a steak with a big bunch of sautéed mushrooms and a pile of spinach.

I decided to try a recipe for shrimp zucchini noodles I found on a Keto Facebook group. My recipe didn't have any actual amounts so I had to guess, but oh my goodness it was good.

Here is the recipe: Shrimp zucchini noodles
Fast and tasty! Sizzle shrimp with garlic and bacon; add heavy cream, Parmesan, salt and pepper to taste. When the sauce starts to get creamy, add spinach and zucchini noodles! Cook it for 1 min and that's it!

I ate half and I saved the other half for tomorrow.

It really is fun trying different recipes and there are so many great Keto options to try.

Day 55 –
I would like to share that I do not like blood work. I usually feel slightly nauseous just thinking about it, and add the fact that I was not able to have anything to eat or drink, not even my half-cup of coffee and you can tell I was a sad, grumpy person. It should take a few days at least to get the results from my doctor, but I do think it's important to get regular physicals, especially if you are doing an extreme low carb diet like Keto.

Needless to say I did not eat or drink anything this morning. When I finally got home I had my coffee and one of the yummy pecan pie fat bombs.
In the afternoon I had my yummy leftovers from yesterday. Peter said he wants to try that recipe using chicken because he is not a big fan of shrimp. I am sure it would be good.

I am facing the next BIG challenge for my weight loss journey; I am flying out today to go visit my daughter and my amazing grandson. It will be difficult to stick with all of my routines when I am not at home, but my daughter has been very supportive. I am sure I can make the best of it. I am bringing my daily food journal so I can continue to keep myself accountable, but I won't have the option of going to work out at the YMCA for the week I am there. I will however be running around with my almost 2 year old grandson so I think that should keep me sufficiently busy.

I had to head to the airport a bit early to accommodate Peter's work schedule, so I had a big chop salad and even treated myself to a beer while at the airport waiting for my flight. Michelob Ultra has only 2.6 carbs so I felt okay treating myself.

I am sad to report that Southwest airlines no longer serves peanuts in case anyone has a peanut allergy, so I wasn't able to have any of the snacks offered, pretzels and crackers are definitely not Keto. I will have to plan ahead for future flights.

Day 56 –
Visiting my daughter will be an interesting challenge to my Keto journey. I started today with some coffee, and I used regular creamer so I am sure that had more carbs than I have been getting, but since I only have one cup of coffee a day I don't think it will be a big problem.

After my adorable grandson woke up, we both had a cheese stick. He enjoyed eating the same thing as grandma. Later I made myself a plate of some turkey lunchmeat with some cheese and some pecans. It was a perfect amount to fill me up for the rest of the day.
My daughter has lots of goodies around the house, including cookies and chips, so there is a lot more temptation, but I am staying strong.
I was so happy to be able to fit more comfortably in the airplane seat yesterday so that gives me more motivation to stick with it.

My daughter was so sweet, she was worried about helping me stick to my diet, but I told her to just cook like normal and I would be able to make it work. I know she is a little skeptical of the diet just like I was, but it is working.

For dinner roasted some cauliflower and she grilled some of those yummy Aidelle's sausages. She also made some corn on the cob, but I let her know I could not have one.

It was a great Keto dinner, except that I of course did not have a bun with my sausage or the corn on the cob.

I won't be able to go workout this week, but hopefully I can take a few walks with William.

Day 57 –
I got a call from my doctor today to report that all my blood work came out great, including my lipids, so no worries about any complications from our diet. That is good news.

I spent the day having fun with my grandson. I started my day with some coffee and we both shared a cheese stick again. We took a fun walk through the neighborhood, stopping to look at every single rock. Walking with a toddler is certainly not a strenuous walk, but it was hot and humid out so we both came inside after our walk and got a big drink of water.

I made us some scrambled eggs with cheese, I ate mine but my grandson only took a few bites of his. Toddlers are so interesting in their eating habits.

We played all afternoon and then he finally took a nap. By the time he woke up my daughter had returned from work so we went out to a meet and greet event. There were lots of delicious homemade goodies, but sadly everything was full of carbs, from yummy little sandwiches to very moist looking brownies. My grandson enjoyed sampling everything, but I just had a small glass of wine.

After we got home my daughter made homemade lettuce wraps. She serves them on a bed of lettuce instead of trying to use the lettuce as an actual wrap. There was some sugar in one of the ingredients, but not enough that I felt like it was a problem to have some.

My grandson decided to help me eat my dinner, so that is another way to control portions; sharing with a small person who is helping himself to your plate.

It's not as completely Keto as I do at home, but so far I am managing pretty well.

Day 58 –
There are so many excuses when it comes to dieting – I know because I used all of them, but I am excited right now because I have stopped using excuses and I am continuing to see results. It is hard and there are times I feel frustrated at the very slow pace of weight loss, but every small victory gives me hope and motivation to continue.

I have been having so much fun playing with my grandson the past few days. We get so busy playing that I hardly have time to think about eating. Today I made scrambled eggs again for breakfast, this time I included chunks of ham that my daughter bought for me, but he was still not interested in eating any. My son-in-law thought it was good though.

We were so busy playing today; riding his tricycle, or rather grandma pushing him on his tricycle, blowing bubbles, hiding under a blanket together, coloring, reading books, and watching his favorite new show Aquanots. I did manage to eat a handful of pecans after he went down for this nap, but then I jumped in the shower and my daughter got home so when he woke up we all went out to dinner.

My daughter was worried about where to go, but I assured her I would be fine almost anywhere. While there are a few obvious places to avoid, like pizza, unless they have the wonderful cauliflower crust that our local place has, or Italian with all the pasta, or even sushi because of the rice, most restaurants can be very Keto-friendly.

We chose a fun place that had a basic menu of burgers, etc. I chose a yummy Black & Blue Burger, which is just a hamburger with blue cheese and bacon. I substituted some broccoli for the fries and removed the bun so I was all set. It was really good and actually a great portion size for me too. I did have a cocktail of some flavored vodka with soda, which is a great low carb alternative.

The hardest part for me was the onion rings. We ordered some onions rings for an appetizer. They smelled so good. I did allow myself a small bite so I wouldn't feel too deprived, and then I was fine. I think those small bites are really helpful. I get to have a 'taste' without really having a portion of something that will throw my whole diet off. It tasted great, but not good enough for me to want to gain back all the weight I've lost. Right now I am making he decisions that will affect my future and getting in shape is more important than a plate of onion rings.

Dinner was fun and because my daughter lives near Nashville, there is great music everywhere. My grandson especially loved the live music.

I have been weighing my self on my daughters scale and although it is slightly off from the YMCA scale at home, I am happy to report that not only have I maintained while on my trip so far, I am even down 1 pound.

Day 59 –
Today was all about family fun and I did not let Keto interfere with any of it. I skipped breakfast, but I did have my usual cup of coffee. I spent the morning playing with my grandson and then when the whole family was ready we went out for a family fun day. We began by picking up some Barbeque. I chose the BBQ Pork and I had some coleslaw as my only side. They included double slaw since a lunch plate includes two sides. I know that BBQ and Coleslaw both usually have some sugar, but I was surprised this one had very little sweet and much more of a spicy kick.

We drove out to a beautiful winery and yes I did sample the wines. I chose the dry or semisweet wines, although they did have a big variety of sweet wines as well. We decided to purchase a couple bottle, one of the reds and one of the sweet whites. My son-in-law and I each had a couple glasses of the red, it was fabulous – it actually is made with some Cajun spices so it tastes a little sweet at first but then you taste the Cajun kick at the end. My daughter was very happy with her sweet peach wine. I know the wine had some carbs but I feel pretty confident I was still well under my carb limit.

We had our picnic and enjoyed our Barbeque and wine and each took turns exploring with my grandson. It was a perfect summer day, sitting in the shade and enjoying each other's company. I think its important to not let Keto be the only focus of your life, enjoying family time together is so important. I have noticed some people online who obsess about their Keto diets; I don't think that is a healthy approach. It might take longer for me to lose weight but life is about balance.

When we were finally ready to leave we actually stopped at another local winery and we sampled there too. I made sure to choose only the dry or semi-sweet wines and the small amount that is included with a sample is not likely to be a large amount of carbs.

We got home and then my daughter made some pork roast and asparagus with Hollandaise sauce. I am still trying to watch my portions but I am not as diligent as I usually am at home. My goal this week is to maintain my weight loss, but if I really want to lose weight I have to be extremely careful with my portions and I know my daughter loves to cook for me and everyone she loves, so I am trying to balance my goals with the goal of enjoying my time here and making her feel happy to take care of her mom. As long as I get home without gaining any weight back I will be happy.

Day 60 -
It was another fun and busy day with my grandson. I got up early with William and I had my coffee and then we played inside and outside.

My daughter made some breakfast sausage and it was a perfect way to start the day.

Several books and coloring pages later we went to a friend's house for a pool party. There were lots of goodies, chips, M&Ms, and really yummy looking brownies, but I just had a few slices of cheese. I know there is nothing keeping me from having goodies except for my personal choice to stick with this diet. It can be hard sometimes, but the desire to lose weight and feel better is more important than the momentary satisfaction of a few chips or a handful of candy. I am happy with the results I am seeing so that keeps me motivated to keep going.

After we got home my son-in-law made amazing shish-kabobs. He had both beef and chicken, and other than a small amount of pineapple, everything on them was perfectly fine for Keto. I had one of each and they were so good. I did splurge and have more of the fantastic wine that we bought the other day.

So far I have been able to keep my diet while here and it hasn't limited my ability to have fun with my family.

Day 61 –
I have been doing a great job trying to stay Keto while at my daughter's house, but I did make one very important exception for today because it is my grandson's second birthday.

I started the day with my coffee and my daughter made some low calories smoothies. We took a fun family trip to the river to go swim and play. My grandson had a blast finding and throwing rocks.

When we got home my daughter made me a fabulous chef salad, with an egg, some ham, turkey and cheese. It was delicious and very filling

After more playtime, my daughter ran out to the store to pick up some things for dinner and for my grandson's special birthday cake.

My daughter was excited to show me what she found at the store. My grandson was having his favorite, Mac-n-cheese for his birthday dinner so she found some vegetable mac-n-cheese for Grandma.

The carbs were a little high, but much lower than regular mac-n-cheese would be and it was so thoughtful of her to try and find a way to include me while keeping me on my diet.

She grilled some burgers and I had some of the veggie version of macaroni. It had a bit of a nutty taste, but overall it wasn't bad.

After dinner we had a fun celebration with an incredible Dirt and Worms cake that my daughter made, and when your 2 year old grandson wants to feed you some of this cake and worms, you eat them – if you are trying to stay on Keto or not. It was really yummy, but definitely not Keto approved.

As much as I want to stick with my diet and lose weight, I also feel very strongly that a diet should not be so restrictive that it interferes with your life and happiness. This diet was supposed to improve my life and health, so an occasion indulgence like birthday cake is not a big deal, and mental health is just as important as physical health.

Day 62 –
Today was my last day of my visit with my daughter and grandson. I made sure to take advantage of every hug and snuggle. We started the morning with my grandson having donuts, which he calls do-do's. Yes, there is temptation to have a donut or two with him, but if I want to have the energy and good health to enjoy playing with him I have to be satisfied with just watching him enjoying his do-dos and he seemed to enjoy his do-do's very much. A little later we both had a cheese stick. He thinks it is fun to eat a cheese stick when I do. Later we played sword fights, we colored and he may have eaten some of a crayon before Grandma let him know that is not food.

I didn't have a lunch because I knew my daughter was planning for us to go out to eat on the way to the airport. Later in the afternoon, after I was all packed and my grandson had finished his nap we all stopped by Outback for one last fun family meal before I left. I do miss having bread, but I knew I had already made a few non-Keto choices during my trip so I did not indulge. I chose a beautiful piece of tilapia with crab meat on top and broccoli and it was great. I knew this meal would be more than enough to keep me full during my flight until I got home.

After a few more hugs and kisses I grabbed my bags and headed to my gate. Even with my weight loss, I am still very large for those very small seats. I was very happy that I could do the seatbelt without too much trouble and no need for an extender. One of the things that I am choosing as a small victory is the fact that I can lower the tray table without it getting stuck on my stomach. This may not seem like much, but for me it is a big improvement.

One of the struggles of being overweight is the internal dialogue that you have with yourself. Despite losing some weight, I know that I am still pretty big and there are times when I feel absolutely enormous. For me airplanes and trying on bathing suits are the worst. It really is a big deal for me to be able to feel like I fit in my seat, even if I still have a long way to go. Celebrating these small victories is a big part of my motivation to continue working hard to lose even more weight.

Day 63 –
Finally home and time to get back on track, but of course since I was gone for a week I have a ton of work to do. I feel bad that I wasn't able to make it to the YMCA today to get back in my exercise groove, but I had two different meetings I had to go to for work, plus lots of laundry and other stuff to get caught up on.

I started my day with my coffee and I grabbed one of the chocolate fat bombs as I rushed out the door to go to my first meeting. It was a breakfast meeting with muffins and fruit, but since I can't have any of that I just tried to appease myself with a big drink from my water bottle.

That meeting took longer than I expected, and I had to leave and go across town for another meeting. I knew that meeting was going to last over 3 hours and that I would be really hungry so I stopped on the way and bought a cheeseburger at McDonalds. When I got it, I took the meat and cheese off the bread and just ate that. I was filling enough to help me get through the afternoon. I know fast food isn't the best choice, but it can be done Keto if you take off the bun and don't have any ketchup. According to Livestrong.com a Quarter pounder with cheese and no bun has between 15 and 20 grams of fat and no carbohydrates at all. I think you can actually order one without the bun, but I didn't think of doing that at the time, so I just took it off the bun and threw the bun away.

I got stuck in traffic on the way home and I was so glad I had packed some pecans in my bags to help me not feel so hungry. When I finally got home I started looking through the fridge, but I had not gone grocery shopping so there wasn't a lot of choices. I decided to cut up some of the Aidelle's sausage and some vegetables. I wanted to make a cream sauce but we didn't have any cream and we didn't have any milk because we haven't been drinking any, so all I had was some sour cream. Well, that failed miserably and Peter and I both threw it in the trash. Sometimes you win, sometimes you learn. We actually laughed about how big a failure that was. I ended up eating a little cheese and a handful of the Crisps that we still had. Peter grilled up something for himself. To top it all off, the kitchen sink got clogged and would not drain – even the garbage disposal hated what I made so now we have to call a plumber.

I will definitely have to go shopping tomorrow.

Day 64 –
I grabbed some coffee this morning and ran out to work. I did manage to pack a lunch of whatever I could find which included a couple cheese sticks, a baggie of pecans and one of the yummy nut rolls. It was boring but it filled me up enough to get through the day.

After work I decided to try and use up more of the remaining food in the fridge. I cooked up the last of an older package of bacon, so Peter and I each had about four pieces each. Next I had a big head of cauliflower so Peter helped and we used the food processor to try and make our own version of cauliflower rice. I used the remaining bacon grease and friend the cauliflower rice but I like the kind at the store much better, the food processor chops great, but the cauliflower comes out too fine and doesn't crisp up quite the same way.

After that Peter joined me and we both made it to the YMCA. I was really happy to get back into my exercise groove. I did about thirty minutes on the treadmill and I felt great. I even stepped up my speed to 3.0. I was so happy that my ankle felt great. My goal is to find time for a workout at least every other day.

Day 65 –
This morning I had my coffee and then I ran out to do a couple errands.

The good news is that I have not gained any weight, but I do seem to be stuck and not losing right now. I have continued to do occasional intermittent fasting in the hopes it will help boost my weight loss again.

After I got home I decided to try a couple fun recipes. First I found a Keto version of Pumpkin Spice. I tried it and to be quite honest it is NOT a good substitute to Starbucks Pumpkin Spice, but it tasted okay.

Next I decided to try a biscuit recipe I found online. There were several sites with very similar variations of this biscuit, but here is the recipe I used.

Low Carb Biscuits Recipe Ingredients
1 1/2 Cups Almond Flour
1/4 Teaspoons Salt
1 Tablespoon Baking Powder
1/2 Teaspoon Garlic Powder
1/2 Teaspoon Onion Powder
2 Eggs
1/2 Cup Sour Cream
4 Tablespoons Butter (melted)
1/2 Cup Shredded Cheddar Cheese

Low Carb Biscuits Recipe Instructions
Preheat the oven to 450 degrees.
Mix the dry ingredient together first.
Combine all the wet ingredients next.
Mix well.
Spray your pan with non-stick cooking spray. Drop a dollop of biscuit batter on your pan. You can also spray the spoon with non-stick cooking spray because the dough will slide right off into the pan. Cook for about 10 to 13 minutes. Serve warm and enjoy!

I used parchment paper instead of cooking spray. These were delicious!!!

I made myself some fried eggs to go with them and it was incredible. Peter tried them when he got home and he loved them too.

I had to work in the afternoon and I was honestly still full when I got home so I decided to just munch on one of the biscuits and skip dinner.

Day 66 –
One again I had another busy, fun-filled day but it was a bit challenging to remain on my Keto diet.

First I ran out to work for a few hours. I did bring along one of those nut bars for a quick breakfast on the go.

After I got home we went over to a friends house for their daughter's birthday party. They had a bunch of birthday treats, including some pizza and cupcakes. Since I hadn't eaten lunch I was hungry. I managed to avoid the cup cakes, but I did have a few pieces of pizza. I am not sure if it impolite, but I simply pulled the cheese topping off of the slices of pizza and ate those. They also had some salad so I had a plate of that too.

Later we went directly from our friend's house to a college football game. It was so hot during the game; Peter and I both were drenched by the end of the first quarter. I did actually have a hot dog at the game, but I tried to pull of most of the bun. It wasn't perfect but I tried to reduce my carbs as much as I could. We have both noticed how much our culture is tied to carbs; popcorn at the movies, hot dogs at the game, pizza with friends, cake for special occasions. All of these make it hard for people who are trying to lose weight. It does take work.

With such a busy day I did not manage to make it to the YMCA, but with all the walking for the football game just to get to our seats I had more than enough steps to feel like I had worked out.

Day 67 –
I had to get up early today to take Peter to the airport. He is traveling for work for two weeks and he is somewhat concerned about being able to make healthy Keto choices while he is traveling. We talked about some of the good healthy options that he can choose. It is not always convenient to diet.

On my way home I stopped at Target and they had Sugar Free Pumpkin Spice Creamer. I don't really care if its actually a good Keto choice or not, I am excited. According to the label it has 2 grams of carbs per one tablespoon serving.

After getting home I worked on some chores and then made myself some tuna fish using my olive oil mayonnaise. I even cut one of the Keto biscuits in half and had a tuna sandwich. I am so happy about those biscuits and I am definitely making them again.

After lunch I went over to the YMCA. I did over 30 minutes on the treadmill and I was able to comfortably walk at the 3.0 speed again. I am feeling really great about working out. While we were walking to and from the football game yesterday I was excited because I could tell I was doing better going up and down stairs. I think the exercise has improved my ankle stability.

After the treadmill, I followed up with about 15 minutes on the stationary bicycle.

The exciting news is that when I went to weigh myself I have now officially reached 20 pounds of weight loss! I do think some of my clothes fit better, and I certainly felt more comfortable when I went on an airplane, but to actually reach 20 pounds feels great! I know I have a lot more to lose but this is a good start.

After I got home I began to think about dinner and with Peter gone I wanted to stick with something simple, but I also had some leftover cauliflower that we had ground up on the food processor. I decided to try and make some mashed cauliflower. I looked online and there are tons of recipes. I found a simple recipe for loaded mashed cauliflower and I basically followed it.
https://www.lowcarbmaven.com/loaded-cauliflower-low-carb-keto/

Since we had already chopped up the cauliflower, I put it in the microwave with some water for about 3-4 minutes.

Next I added that to the mixer with butter, sour cream, salt, pepper, onion and garlic powder and after mixing that for a bit I added some shredded cheddar cheese. It didn't get very fluffy, I think the cauliflower was too wet so I decided to put it in small glass dishes and bake it in the over for about 15-20 minutes. I added some extra cheddar cheese on top because…duh…who doesn't want extra cheddar cheese, and that is what they did in the recipe I looked at. After baking I tried one of the dishes and it was really good. The consistency is not the same as mashed potatoes and I am not sure if that is due to my skills or just the nature of cauliflower. I honestly thought it felt more like grits, but it tasted yummy.

I do love how many new fun food options we have tried or learned about due to this diet.

Day 68 -
I enjoyed my coffee this morning with my sugar free pumpkin spice creamer. I headed straight out to work so I skipped breakfast.

I did pack myself a nice healthy lunch of salad with pumpkin seeds and feta cheese and some Italian dressing.

When I got home I took a few minutes to relax and then made myself a hamburger with one of the mozzarella cheese balls in the middle to make it more fun. It was a perfect dinner.

I was disappointed because I wasn't able to make it to the YMCA today, I had a meeting I had to go to and it lasted longer than I thought so it was too late to go workout after.

Peter called and said he was not making good diet decisions, and he felt bad, but the good news is that he was able to check with the YMCA in Wisconsin and it looks like they may let him swim there so that's good. It is not as much fun as going together but if he keeps up his exercise that would be great.

Day 69-
Another busy day at work, but luckily I planned ahead. I started my day with my coffee & my delicious sugar free pumpkin spice creamer.

I had prepared some awesome chicken salad last night that included chicken, cheese and chopped pecans. It was a perfect lunch.

After work I got to relax for a few minutes, and then I headed out to my monthly book club meeting. The waitress at the wine bar where we usually meet knows that I am on a low carb diet. At our last meeting she let me know that Prosecco has the lowest amount of carbs for all the wines they have, so I had two glasses of Prosecco during our fun meeting. My book club is full of amazing women. I spent the evening laughing and sharing fun stories. I chose to have a cup of the Lobster bisque. I am not sure if it is completely Keto friendly, but it is delicious. They usually serve it with bread, but I just had my soup and my wine, as well as some water and I was fine.

I was not able to go workout today, but I know I walked quite a bit at work, and I will plan to go to the YMCA tomorrow.

I would like to be more consistent with exercise, but sometimes life just gets too busy to make it to the YMCA as often as I would like. I am still feeling really positive overall about our diet and our results so far. I know it I a long journey, but I know we are both making progress toward our goals.

Day 70 –
I started the day with a quick cup of coffee and then headed to work for a few hours. I ran around and did a few errands, including a much-needed trip to the grocery store.

It is hard to always stay motivated and today I really struggled while walking through the grocery aisles. The bread, the chips, the crackers, the cereal – it all seemed to be calling out to me. I filled my cart with so many great things, lots of cheeses and loads of vegetables, but I will admit it is really hard walking by all the things that I shouldn't eat.

When I got home I quickly re-heated my leftover mashed cauliflower. It was still yummy.

Even though Peter is gone, I am still trying to make a good effort to make really healthy Keto dinners, so tonight I used some leftover chicken and made myself the Keto Chicken Enchiladas with rolled cheese shells. They were so good I had four of them.

I was full and feeling lazy and it was hard to motivate myself to get up and go workout, but I knew that I had not been there for the past two nights so I grabbed my tennis shoes and headed to the YMCA. I did my usual 35 minutes on the treadmill and I really can feel that I am getting in better shape, I am able to walk at higher speeds without any ankle or knee pain so that is great. I am looking forward to the weather cooling off just a bit so I can begin to go on walks with my dog again soon.

Seeing positive results on the scale, or the fit of my clothes or being able to handle higher speeds on the treadmill are the kind of things that keep me motivated.

Day 71 –
I was so happy that it was finally a bit cooler this morning. After my coffee I was able to take Lexi on a short walk outside. We only managed about 30 minutes before it was too hot, but she was really excited to get a chance to go sniff around the neighborhood.

After I got back home I decided to make myself some scrambled eggs. My daughter told me to try adding some cottage cheese to my scrambled eggs. She assured me it helps make them fluffier, and since cottage cheese is allowed on Keto I decided to give it a try and I thought they came out great.

I had a bunch of work to do today, but I made a point of getting up every hour or so to walk around, or find and excuse to walk upstairs. I know that Apple watches remind people to get up and move and I think that is a great idea. My fitbit monitors if I have walked at least 250 steps every hour, but it doesn't have the ability to remind me to move. With everyone spending so much time on computers, we all need reminders to move more.

I did have to go to work for a few hours in the afternoon and after I got home I used my leftovers to make more of those delicious chicken enchiladas with cheese shells. They are so good.

I am feeling really positive about how things are going. I know it is getting harder with all the Halloween treats everywhere, but if I stay focused I can keep making good choices and keep losing weight.

Day 72 –
I am really amazed that we have both stuck with our commitment to this diet for 72 days now. Not only that but I have somehow

managed to write a daily blog post for 72 straight days. It is a pretty incredible accomplishment.

Today I had to work so I grabbed my morning coffee and headed out the door.

I had packed myself a very basic lunch with some cucumber and cheese sticks and a container of Crisps. It wasn't exciting but it did fill me up and help me get through the day.

After I got home I decided to try the shrimp and zucchini dish again, but it didn't work out as well this time. I'm not sure what I did differently, except that I didn't start with bacon, I just sautéed the shrimp in butter and garlic. I added the heavy cream and Parmesan, and then I added the zucchini and spinach. I might have used too much spinach? Or I might not have let the cream sauce thicken enough, but it came out very watery. I tried to add a bit more Parmesan and it didn't really melt, it just clumped up together. Overall it tasted okay but definitely not as good as the first time I made it.

I did decide to have some dark chocolate after dinner. I have a chocolate bar that says it is only 14 carbs for 12 squares of chocolate. Sometimes you just need some chocolate, and on a Friday after a long week I decided to splurge. I knew I was pretty low for my overall carbs today so I felt comfortable allowing myself the indulgence.

I did not go workout today. Honestly I was tired from a long week and just wanted to curl up and read a book. I think its okay to give yourself permission to relax. Being able to read your body signals is important and I will find time to exercise this weekend. I am planning to check out a yoga class, which is a bit intimidating for me. It is hard for overweight people to do yoga so this is a big challenge for me, but after doing Keto for the past 72 days my confidence in growing and I know I can handle it.

Day 73 –

I feel like I do much better during the week because weekends tend to have more social activities and much more opportunity to struggle with staying Keto.

This morning I got up and had my coffee and began doing some chores around the house. Sometime in the mid-morning I had one of he chocolate fat bombs that we made. I am not entirely sure how long they can last but it was still good.

Later I had to go over to work for a little while, and after that I was hungry so I stopped at a McDonalds drive through and ordered a plain quarter pounder with cheese. I removed the bun and just ate the burger patty. It is surprising how that actually does satiate you enough to make it until dinner.

Immediately after I went to a fun political event. It was a mixer and a rally. I enjoyed sitting with friends and learning more about the important issues and candidates. I was planning to go right home after the event, but my friends asked if I would go with them to a local brewery that was only a block from where we were. It's a place I really like so I relented and decided to join them.

It was a struggle to stay Keto because there were no low carb beer options and this brewery makes really great beer so I decided to indulge and had an Octoberfest. It tasted amazing. We all chose something to eat. I was considering wings because the waitress assured me the wings there are not breaded but I decided on a Cobb style salad. The only challenge was that the salad was topped with friend chicken, which was breaded. I did try to avoid eating as much breading as I could, but basically my meal was not exactly Keto. It was however delicious.

Despite not being perfect, I am still doing well on the scale, slowly going down by just a little bit each day. I have not been to the YMCA for a couple days, but it's okay. I have been active and busy so that helps.

Having stuck with this diet for 73 days now with only minor cheat episodes I still feel pretty good about our accomplishments. This isn't a sprint, it's a marathon and at this point I am working on how to really incorporate our new low carb lifestyle in a way that is healthy and sustainable so we can ultimately reach our goal weights.

Day 74 -
Today was another day where I tried my best to stay Keto, but I was not perfect.

After being woken up early by my husband who is on the east coast and really excited about attending the Packers football game, I got up and had my coffee. I checked and saw the game was not televised on regular TV so I decided to head over to our local sports bar to watch the game.

I decided to have some breakfast and although they had a bunch of choices that were not Keto, I ordered just some scrambled eggs and bacon. Even that was served with a big container of ketchup that I did not use.

Although I wanted some other fun choices of beer I decided to stick with a very low carb choice of Michelob Ultra with only 2.6 carbs in a bottle.

After halftime I did splurge and order myself some Queso dip with pork, but I asked for veggies instead of chips. Even that choice is a challenge because carrots have a lot of sugar and thus a lot of carbs so I did not eat them, and I will admit queso does not taste the same with celery.

I looked up how many carbs in tortilla chips and asked the waitress if she could bring me just a few chips and I ate about 5-6 chips. It was just enough to really enjoy them, and I broke them into smaller pieces so I could feel like I had more than I actually did.

The game went into overtime and honestly I was so tired by the time I got home that actually took a nap. That might have something to do with how early my hubby woke me up. Anyway for dinner I finished off my leftover shrimp and zucchini dish.

I am actually happy to get back to the workweek tomorrow so I can get back into my more healthy routines.

Even though I have made a commitment to 100 full days of Keto, I am starting to think more about long terms lifestyle changes so I can maintain my current weight loss and continue losing weight. That is why I am not being overly strict with my Keto every single day, but just focusing on making good choices and trying to stay within my daily carb limit of 25 carbs or less. Eventually I will feel comfortable raising that limit, but for now I am still continuing to lose so I will continue to limit my daily carbs.

Day 75 –
Wow - I am ¾ done with my 100 days! That is pretty impressive. This morning I grabbed some coffee and ran out the door to go to work. I packed a really quick and light lunch, once again including a cut up cucumber and a couple cheese sticks. After over-doing it during the weekend I wanted to get back to my healthier choices and portions. I had one of the nut bars for an afternoon snack.

When I got home I finished up some chores and then made myself a healthy dinner. I started with a couple chicken breasts. I made up a mixture of mayonnaise (about 2 tablespoons) and spices (salt, pepper, garlic, onion and Penzies Italian seasoning) and then added some shredded Parmesan cheese. I mixed all of those together and put a spoonful on top of each chicken breast, which I then baked at 375 for about 30 minutes. While that was cooking I cooked some cauliflower rice in a pan until crispy. I always add some garlic to the butter as I am cooking, to give the cauliflower more flavor.

I was hungry and it tasted great. After dinner I decided to head over to the YMCA to go workout. I had already walked a ton at work so I decided to focus on the stationary bicycle and I rode for a little about 40 minutes while I listened to an audio book.

I did walk a bit more and actually made my 10,000 step daily goal so my fitbit sent happy green notifications. One of the things that I noticed was moving at least 250 steps every single hour except one.

I did talk with Peter about possibly getting an Apple watch at some point in the future. I do like my basic fitbit, but there are some cool functions available on the Apple watch that I don't currently have, like reminders to get up and move when I have been sitting too long, and the new Apple watch does amazing things regarding monitoring your heart rate.

I watched an incredible video on Facebook today that discussed how great exercise is for your mind, not just your body so that just made me more motivated to keep on exercising.

https://www.facebook.com/TED/videos/10160545401360652/

Every single day it is a choice to eat right and exercise and some days those choices are much harder than others, but I am excited about the results so far and that helps to keep me on track.

Day 76 –
After grabbing a quick coffee to go, I jumped in the car and headed out. I went to work outside this morning and it got hot fast. Although I brought my water bottle with me I quickly finished all that and was extremely grateful when one of the women I was working with had more nice cold water for us.

Once I got home I cooled off, drank a Gatorade (the ones with zero calories) and more water and then made myself a quick lunch of egg salad.
Then I headed over to my brother and sister-in-laws's house to go hang out with my dad so they could have some time to themselves. They were so sweet and made sure to let me know they had plenty of Keto friendly food in the house. It really helps when you have supportive family and friends; it makes a big difference when trying to lose weight.

I got some work done while Dad was hanging out watching TV, and when it was time for dinner I gave him some options. He decided to have some leftover pork roast that my sister-in-law had made. I fixed up some rice for Dad and warmed up some of the pork. I decided to have some leftover broccoli and cheese with a little of the pork.

I try to help out my brother and sister-in-law as often as I can and come over to stay with Dad. They do such a great job taking care of Dad, so coming over once in awhile so they can have a night away seems like the least I can do. I also just like getting the chance to talk with Dad. He is 89 years old and he is still so sharp, unfortunately his body is no longer cooperating the way it used to. We have fun conversations about the joys of grandchildren, and he shares funny stories from his past. This time together is so valuable to me.

When I finally made it home I was exhausted, but I felt good because I know I did a good job of sticking with my diet today. Each and every day on Keto is a matter of deciding to do what's best for your long-term health and it isn't always easy, but I do think it is worth it.

Day 77 –
I finally had a day to just relax and catch up on all the things I have needed to get done. I started my day with my usual coffee. It was cloudy out and I even treated myself to a second cup of coffee. After working on the computer for a couple hours I decided to go ahead and try another Keto recipe. I made myself 'cheese buns' from a recipe I found.

There were very few ingredients and it seemed weird to just mix the egg in with the cheese, but I stirred until I felt like it was evenly and thoroughly coated.

I put the two piles of the mixture onto parchment paper and slid the pan into the oven.

I was concerned that 20 minutes at 400 degrees sounded like a lot and I thought it might burn so I checked a few times and it seemed to be doing great.

They tasted good, but very cheesy. The outside was a bit tough, but inside it actually had a somewhat fluffy almost bread-like texture.

It was so nice and cool out after the rain that I decided to take Lexi for a long walk rather than head over to the YMCA. We waked for about 40 minutes and she was so excited to be out sniffing every bush that we actually kept a pretty brisk pace. It was a good workout.

After we got home I re-heated some of the leftover chicken from yesterday and threw some cauliflower rice into a pan to crisp. When it was golden brown and crispy I actually added about a tablespoon of Parmesan cheese on top and stirred it in to melt. It really added a nice touch to the rice.

I am feeling good about my diet choices lately so I am hoping that will continue to translate to lower numbers on the scale.

Day 78 –
I grabbed my coffee and headed out this morning, but luckily I only had to work for a few hours. I had one of the Nut Bars for a morning snack, and when I made it home I heated up the last of the leftover chicken for my lunch.

I decided to try another new recipe for dinner. I spiralized two zucchinis and set them out to dry for a while.

Here is the recipe:
Ingredients
- 4 Zucchinis
- 1/2 stick of butter
- 2 cloves of garlic
- 1 cup parmesan cheese
- salt

Instructions
1 Turn zucchini into noodles using a julienne peeler, spiralizer or
        veggetti.
2 Put zucchini noodles into a colander and salt liberally let sit for 20
        minutes (very important!)
3 After 20 minutes, rinse and pat dry with a paper towel
4 Melt butter and the garlic in a skillet or sauté pan
5 Sauté noodles over med-high heat for 4-5 minutes
Remove from heat and mix in Parmesan cheese

*for the recipe check this website:
https://www.almostsupermom.com/one-skillet-garlic-parmesan-
zoodles/

This is how the Zoodles looked on the website

This is how my dish came out – not quite the pretty dish they
showed. My cheese melted too much and I had a lot of moisture in
my pan, but they tasted great.

I actually ate too much because it was so yummy and I was hungry,
so after dinner I really didn't feel like going to workout. I laid on the
sofa and snuggled with my dog while watching TV for a while but
after an hour I decided that whether I feel like it or not, I need to go
workout so I headed to the YMCA.

I started on the treadmill and walked for a little over 30 minutes.

Then I did the stationary bicycle for another 10 minutes.

I have tried to make sure my workouts are at least 35-45 minutes
long.

I decided to go check my weight since it had been a while since I
checked and …..

I have now lost a total of 21 pounds! I was hoping that it would be
more, but it is still a great number.

Day 79 –
Blogging each day for 79 straight days has been quite a commitment, but I feel like my commitment to blogging has helped to keep me accountable. Even though it's late I did manage to find a few minutes to get my blog posted today. It's getting harder to find original ways to share what I did and ate each day.

This morning I grabbed some coffee and headed out to work. We didn't have much in the ay of lunch food so I just had to make do. I grabbed a couple cheese sticks, some pecans and a small container of Crisps, but it was enough to get me through the day. When I got home I made a late lunch of steamed broccoli and a piece of lemon-butter fish.

I stopped at a quick Democratic house party and then went to pick Peter up at the airport. I knew Peter had not had the chance to eat any dinner so I asked him if he wanted to stop and get some of that delicious cauliflower crust pizza. He said yes immediately.

I did not really need any pizza, but I enjoyed my date night with Peter who was finally home after two weeks. We ate and enjoyed each bite as we listened to some really awful Karaoke.

Peter said he did not do a good job of sticking with Keto while he was away so he was very happy to be home and he has committed to getting back to making good diet choices now that he is back home.

I really am lucky to be able to do this together with Peter. Being able to encourage and support each other has been incredible.

Day 80 –
While I didn't make it around the world, for the past 80 days I have stuck with the Keto diet and with just a couple rare exceptions I have stayed very true to this diet. I had hoped that my weight loss to this point might be much bigger, but I am pleased overall at my results.

With only twenty days left of my 100-day commitment I have every
confidence that I will finish strong.

Today, along with my coffee, I started my day with a big breakfast
of bacon and scrambled eggs. Peter tends to put way too much food
on my plate, so I only ate about half of the eggs he gave me. We all
have to learn that it is OKAY to not finish all the food on your plate.
If you are full STOP EATING.

After breakfast I jumped in the car to attend an all day Democratic
state meeting, which was over 2 hours away. I was still full from the
big breakfast so I did not have lunch when I got there. I also did not
get the lunch because there was very little of it I could actually eat
since it consisted of a big sandwich and a bag of chips.
I also had to decline when friends offered cookies and other snacks
they had packed for the meeting. I don't want to be rude, but my
health is more important than worrying if someone will be upset that
I don't want their kindly offered snacks.

Fortunately the meeting didn't last too long and I was on my way
back home by 4:00. I was a bit hungry at that point so I went ahead
and stopped at fast food, ordering a cheeseburger of which I ate only
the patty, and threw away the buns. It was enough to get me through
the drive home.

For dinner I ate the second half of a big burger Peter had made for
himself with mozzarella cheese inside. I also made myself some
steamed broccoli to go with it.

I rarely do this, but since it was a weekend I treated myself to a small
bowl of the low carb ice cream that I bought for Peter. Its okay to
have dessert once in awhile, especially if it is a good choice like this
low carb ice cream.

I did not get a chance to go workout today, but I will make time for a
visit to the YMCA tomorrow.

Day 81 –

Weekends can be great for diets but they can also be full of struggles. After a relaxing morning with my coffee, Peter and I went out to the grocery store and then came home to watch football on TV.

I found these fun drinks at the store and decided these would be a good alternative to beer or wine while watching the game.

They taste great and they are only 2 carbs for the whole can.

Peter decided to make bratwurst and we also made some Sauerkraut, which is very low in carbs. Other than the bun this is exactly what we would be having on any normal football Sunday, so staying Keto isn't that difficult.

The biggest problem for me is that I really wanted to eat some chips. I really miss chips, especially while watching a game. I decided to make myself some cheese 'chips' and while they did taste good they were not quite the chip feeling that I was longing for. For me, the hardest part of Keto is not having crunchy foods like chips, pretzels and crackers that I love. I do use nuts for crunch but it is something I really miss.

To make these cheese chips just take a small amount of cheese into piles on some parchment paper and bake at 400 degrees for approximately 5-6 minutes. My chips came out a bit large but you can make them any size that you want.

After the game we watched a movie together and I was so tired from getting up several times during the night with my dog that wasn't feeling well so I actually fell asleep and I slept through dinner. I guess that is one way to do an intermittent fast.

Needless to say I did not make it to the YMCA, but I really needed the sleep and sleep is incredibly important for weight loss.

Day 82 –
I grabbed my coffee this morning and headed out for a busy day.

After attending a meeting this morning I had a few minutes to grab some lunch before working all afternoon. I decided to stop at a cool place called *Salad and Go.* I ordered a big Cobb salad but asked for no tomatoes to stay Keto. The salad was fantastic. With bacon, avocado, egg, and lots of fresh greens it was a perfect Keto lunch.

After getting home Peter and I cooked dinner together. He really wanted to make the Keto Chicken Enchiladas with the cheese shells. They are so yummy. I actually had a second helping.

Even though I had gotten a lot of sleep yesterday I was really tired after dinner. I'm not sure if it is allergies or something else, but I have been so busy lately and I think my body just needs some recuperation time. I really believe it's important to listen to your body.

As I get closer to the end of my 100 days I am thinking about how we will both continue to focus on a low carb diet to continue our weight loss journey.

Day 83 –
Although my schedule is pretty hectic, I do try to schedule at least one day a week where I can stay home and catch up on dishes, laundry, chores, etc. Today was my day to stay home, or at least I was hoping it would be.

I took my time enjoying my coffee and mid-morning I decided to make myself a healthy breakfast. I cut up some ham and made myself some scrambled eggs with ham and cheese. I mixed a tablespoon of cottage cheese in with my eggs and it came out fluffy and great. I only used 2 eggs but it looked like much more.

I worked on chores; laundry, dishes, etc. and I got the chance to focus on some office work and phone calls. I wound up with a last minute appointment however, so I had to run upstairs and jump in the shower to make it on time.

After work I met with one of my fabulous friends to plan our upcoming trip to Thailand. I am so excited. I can absolutely guarantee that I will not be worrying about staying Keto while in Thailand. Part of the adventure of traveling is eating all the unique foods from that area. I am not overly concerned about gaining a bunch of weight because travel also involves a lot of walking and activity.

I did order a fantastic salad and although it had some small cut up pieces of pear, everything else in the salad was Keto friendly, as well as delicious.

When I got home I relaxed with Peter and treated myself to a small amount of dark chocolate, he helped himself to a bowl of the low carb ice cream. I really do believe these small indulgences are what keep us doing so well on our diet. I am much less likely to need to 'cheat' when I allow myself to have a treat once in awhile, and these treats are appropriately low in carbs.

Not only that, but chocolate, especially dark chocolate has a whole bunch of health benefits.

7 Proven Health Benefits of Dark Chocolate
- Very Nutritious.
- Powerful Source of Antioxidants.
- May Improve Blood Flow and Lower Blood Pressure.
- Raises HDL and Protects LDL From Oxidation.
- May Reduce Heart Disease Risk.
- May Protect Your Skin From the Sun.
- Could Improve Brain Function

For more info check out this blog post
https://www.healthline.com/nutrition/7-health-benefits-dark-chocolate

I do need to be more consistent with exercise, but life always seems to throw a curve ball. I had planned to exercise in the afternoon but then wound up with a last minute work thing. I know that is an excuse and I could wake up early and exercise or find another time to go. I like when I can build exercise into my normal activity, but it really is up to me to MAKE myself commit to go to the YMCA at least every other day, especially if I want to be in good shape for my upcoming trip.

Day 84 –
I enjoyed my coffee this morning. I am almost out of my sugar free pumpkin spice creamer so I will have to get some more soon. It really makes my morning coffee feel like a special treat.

I was happy to have the day off today so later in the morning I decide to make more of the Keto biscuits Peter had been asking for.

The biscuits are easy to make, just a few ingredients. For the recipe visit my previous blog post http://meandmychubbyadventures.blogspot.com/2018/09/our-keto-journey-day-65.html

 I had two of the biscuits when they were warm and they tasted so good. I saved the rest for later. I just threw them in a baggie and tossed them in the fridge.

I got lots of work done and just grabbed a cheese stick for a quick lunchtime snack.

After Peter got home I made some salmon while he grilled a steak and we had green beans.

After dinner I ran out to a meeting for a couple hours and when I got home I watched a little TV until I was ready for bed. I did indulge myself again with a couple of the remaining squares of chocolate.

I felt bad that I didn't manage time to get to the YMCA, but I felt good about my diet choices.

Day 85 –
It was another extremely crazy busy day. After grabbing some coffee
I quickly packed a lunch and headed out to work.

I packed some pecans, a couple cheese sticks and a quick salad with
some spinach and pumpkin seeds. It wasn't exciting but it was edible
and it was enough to get me through the day.

When I got home I grabbed the leftover salmon and re-heated it and
it was just right.

Peter called and I met him at the Verizon store to upgrade my phone.
That took awhile and I headed straight from there to a meeting I had,
which of course lasted longer than I expected.

When I got home I was exhausted and Peter made a comment about
how he wised he could have a big glass of milk, but he can't. Then
he said he can't ever have milk again and I had a meltdown. It was
all just too much for me today. I know it was because I was tired, but
I came a bit unglued, letting him know that when he says things like
that it will cause me to fail on this diet. If I believe that I cant EVER
have chips, or milk, or whatever I know that will be too hard for me
and it will cause me to fail.

I made this commitment to 100 days and so far I have been able to
keep it, but I am really at the point where I am frustrated at not
losing more and getting really tired of the deprivation I feel.
This is the greatest challenge with any diet. According to
sharecare.com "Diets fail for the very same psychological reasons
that cause us to overeat. They are dependent on an unhealthy
relationship with eating. In one case we over eat to excess not to
meet the physical needs of hunger but to meet the emotional
demands of life."

Obsessing over food is the problem. Either obsessing over it and
eating too much or obsessing over it and restricting are both still a

problem because it is an unhealthy relationship with food. Research shows that even after losing weight, people often will struggle to keep that weight off.

There is a great deal of information on why and how diets don't work. This article in Self magazine was very good. https://www.self.com/story/why-diets-fail

I don't want everyone to think I am sabotaging my diet or giving up, quite the contrary. I know that when I focus on unhealthy attitudes like restriction of foods, especially when I make fatalistic statements like I can 'Never have that again" that I am making choices that will absolutely lead to failure.

I made a commitment to do a "diet" for 100 days and I have just over two weeks left in that commitment, but I still have a lot of weight to lose and more importantly I still need to work on improving my health and fitness level. Once my 100 days are finished I will still need to "incorporate lots of physical activity, be extremely mindful of my diet and hunger cues, and manage stress without relying on food", as the author of the Self article indicated. I still do believe that diets do not work, but a commitment to health and choosing healthy practices can work. Reframing my language and self-talk is the key to success.

Day 86 –
I started my day with my usual cup of coffee. I know that many people on Keto do intermittent fasting and that according to most Keto websites you should only have black coffee or water during the hours you are fasting, but although I am limiting my eating to only 8 hours in the day, I am just not willing to give up my creamer.

After finishing some paperwork in the morning I grabbed a couple cheese sticks and a cut up cucumber for my lunch and headed out to work. My diet has been fairly boring and basic, but it does seem to be working. The scale is continuing to slowly inch down.

After working in the afternoon and struggling through a lengthy commute in traffic I met some friends for a fun evening out. I chose a delicious chicken and pecan salad and had a glass of Prosecco. According to Yummywineblog.com Champagne and other sparkling wines like brut or prosecco have around 98 calories and 1.5g of carbs for a 5oz serving, which makes them the best wines to drink if you're watching calories or carbs!

Only two more weeks of my 100 day commitment and even though I am getting bored and tired of dieting and of writing these daily blog posts, I am excited to be nearing the end of this commitment.

Day 87 –
Today was not a good day. It started out okay. I had my coffee. I had to work for a couple hours.

When I got home I made myself a nice healthy chicken salad.

That's when it started to take a turn downhill. My husband and I got ready to attend a football game. We put on our college colors and headed out the door. It was hot out. There was so much fun college atmosphere in the air. We were both really tired of our diet.

My first bad choice was to have a regular beer, not a low carb one. I checked online and they have 6.5 carbs, so not terrible but that isn't where our evening ended.

When we got to the game we walked up to the snack bar and all I could see and smell was the yummy popcorn. It has been so long since I've had popcorn. Peter had two regular hot dugs, and yes that was with the bun and all. I thought I was being smart and would get the bratwurst. Well it wasn't very good, boiled not grilled and despite removing a bunch of the bun I did eat probably 1/3 of the bun. A quick check indicates that a hot dog bun is about 21 carbs so I would guess I ate 8-10 carbs.

Sitting in the stands watching the game Peter asked if I wanted anything else and I blurted out – "Yes I want popcorn". I knew I shouldn't but I really wanted some. Despite doing so well on the diet I just wanted the sweet, salty crunchy feel of popcorn. Peter came back to our seats with a big bucket of popcorn. We both had a bunch and I enjoyed it, all the while feeling guilty for allowing myself the indulgence. There are 21 grams of carbs in ONE ounce of popcorn, so needless to say we were way over our limit for today.

I think being so close to the end of my 100-day commitment has me feeling a sense of frustration for these 100 days to be over already. Even with this poor choice today, I have been consistent on this diet. I know that once night of a few too many carbs from a beer and some popcorn is not the end of the world, but the concern is that allowing myself one indulgence could lead to another…and another and all my hard work could vanish. I will not do that. I will get back to my good eating choices and keep working hard to get the weight off.

Day 88 –
Trying to negotiate staying on Keto with still being able to enjoy the typical weekend fun that we usually participate in can be tricky. I am really trying to see how I can still do all the activities I enjoy, but make them more Keto friendly. I know that being able to do this will mean that I can actually continue a low carb diet for long-term weight loss.

Today we did just that. We went to one of our favorite sports bars to go watch NFL football. Typically football Sundays involve drinking and often some not as healthy foods and snacks.

I started with a yummy breakfast wrap, but because a tortilla shell has about 15 total carbs I removed as much excess from the tortilla that I reasonably could. I know I could just order scrambled eggs, but I am honestly tired of just having scrambled eggs and I am trying to find possible low carb alternatives that I can eat. I probably only ate half of the tortilla.

At halftime I decided to get some wings. Fortunately these wings are not breaded so they are Keto friendly. I also made sure to ask for all celery and no carrots with my wings.

I did decide to have a mimosa but I made sure to have it very light on orange juice so it was basically champagne, which has very few carbs.

Later that night I made myself some zoodles with alfredo sauce.

I am not sure why it came out different but the sauce was really thick this time; it tasted great though.

Day 89 –
Even though Peter and I are almost finished with our 100 day commitment, we have both decided that we will continue a low carb lifestyle until we are able to lose enough weight to come close to our goal, but I will not continue to do daily blog posts. I might continue with monthly updates on our weight loss so far.

This morning I grabbed some coffee and headed out to work. One of the part time jobs I have is to lead field trips around the Botanical Gardens. The gardens are beautiful, it is a great way to get some exercise and I love being with the students as they learn about and explore the garden. Today was our orientation meeting for the new season of the garden. The head of our department was so sweet; she got a bunch of amazing goodies for everyone to eat before we got started. There were so many yummy looking goodies including chocolate and crème-filled Danish and the most adorable little cupcakes with little desert plants made from green icing decorating the top of the cupcakes. I so wanted to eat some but I knew that it would not get me to my goals.

It is hard to refrain from having "just one" but I know those carbs will not help me to achieve my goals. I just had my cup of coffee and appreciated how pretty the snacks all were. There is no question that this is the hardest part of 'dieting'. I could have chosen to take a small Danish and just have one bite. Sometimes that is a good choice

so you don't feel so deprived. Being able to deal with temptation
and make healthy choices is the hardest part of any weight loss goal.

The meeting only lasted for the morning so I came home and
grabbed one of the last remaining Keto biscuits in the fridge and
some cheese. It was a great snack to keep me going. Later I cup up a
cucumber. I love cucumbers and they are a great low carb source of
nutrients and fiber.
After Peter got home we worked together to make the stuffed
peppers that he wanted to try.

I found a basic recipe online.

We started by cutting up some onion and garlic and sautéing them in
a pan. Next we added the cauliflower rice to help that get softened
and add flavor. Next we added some ground beef, along with some
seasoning of salt, pepper, garlic powder and onion powder. When
the ground beef was no longer pink we added some tomato sauce
and let it simmer for just a little bit.

While Peter was working on the inside, I grabbed some beautiful
peppers we got at the grocery store and cut off the tops, cleaning out
the inside. The recipe said to put some salt and pepper inside the
peppers so I did.

We carefully filled each pepper with the mixture and left some room
at the top, which we covered with a generous amount of mozzarella
cheese. Peter is a Wisconsin boy, so anything that we can put cheese
on he is very happy. The recipe said to keep the tops on while
cooking but we decided we wanted to top them with cheese instead.
They were delicious.

I love looking up new healthy recipes and cooking with Peter. This
makes our whole Keto journey more interesting and the variety helps
us do a better job of sticking to our diet.

Day 90 –

Today was a cool rainy day so it seemed perfect for a crockpot recipe.

I read comments from several people online in my Keto groups talking about something called Crack Chicken so I decided I had to give it a try. Here is link to the recipe I found.
 http://fitmomjourney.com/slow-cooker-crack-chicken/

Slow Cooker Crack Chicken

I'm not kidding when I tell you this magical fact about Slow Cooker Crack Chicken:

It takes 4 ingredients and less than 5 minutes to put together.

It's super simple to make:

Put 4 chicken breasts in the bottom of a (linked) slow cooker. It's totally ok for them to be completely, totally frozen. Keep it easy.

Dump 2 packets of ranch dressing mix over the chicken breasts.

Then place 2 blocks of cream cheese on top of the chicken.

Set the slow cooker to low for 8 hours, then hustle out the door to work & school.

When it's almost time to serve the Crack Chicken, microwave some bacon, crumble it, and stir it in. Bonus points if you also microwave a broccoli steamer to serve the Slow Cooker Crack Chicken over.

It was very easy; I put the chicken in the crockpot, covered it with the seasoning packets and put the cream cheese on top and turned it on. I love crockpot cooking, just set it and forget it.

While the chicken was cooking I decided to make myself some breakfast, or more accurately some brunch since it was after 11:00am. I followed the instructions and once again made two cheese buns (the recipe with half cup of mozzarella cheese and one egg). I also made myself a fried egg to go with it.
After about 4 hours I did open the crockpot to check on the dish and since the cream cheese was still basically in large chunks on top of the chicken I did stir it around a bit to ensure that it melted properly. When Peter got home we fried up some cauliflower rice and served the chicken over rice. It was VERY thick and creamy but it tasted delicious. Peter was a big fan.

There are a lot of great Keto alternatives for meals.

Day 91 –
Wow, it really does feel impressive to be on day 91. I am a bit frustrated because I feel like my weight is not only NOT going down right now, but it actually went back up two pounds. I could understand after our 'cheating' last weekend, but I have been so careful for the past 3-4 days and it still isn't moving down. I am wondering if maybe there is a hormonal reason for being stuck. Even though I am technically in menopause, I do know that I still have an occasional episode of retaining water, craving carbs and feeling grumpy. This might be the reason I am stuck this week.

Today I started with my usual coffee. I was actually hungry at work this morning, but luckily I had planned for that and I had brought one of the health nut bars. It was a perfect option to keep me going until lunch. I only had to work half a day so when I came home I cooked up the leftover zoodles with alfredo sauce. I added some spinach in for even more veggie goodness with nutrients and fiber.

For dinner Peter and I both had some leftovers. I re-heated some of the crack chicken and made some fresh broccoli to go with it. At first

Peter didn't want any broccoli but he decided to have some and even said it came out great. I am really working hard to ALWAYS include veggies with our meals.

After dinner I asked Peter to help 'force me' to go to the YMCA. It is so easy to feel 'too tired' after a busy day and I let him know I need his help and support to get there. This is still an area that we struggle with. I know I always feel better after I go, but sometimes it is just so hard to make myself get out the door. Going together has really helped quite a bit.

I managed to do my 30+ minutes on the treadmill and I pushed myself to walk at 3.0 speed so it was a good workout.

The really big news is that despite my slight bump in weight for the past two days on my home scale, I checked on the YMCA scale and I have lost a total of 30 pounds since we started our Keto journey.

That is an average of 10 pounds per month, which is really encouraging, and it makes me feel like I really can reach my goal weight.

Day 92 –
I had a chance to stop by Target yesterday so this morning I got to enjoy my cup of coffee with sugar free pumpkin spice creamer. The mornings are finally starting to cool off so it really helps to feel like fall when I can relax and enjoy my coffee with pumpkin spice and still stay relatively Keto friendly.

I did have to go to work for a few hours and when I got home I finished up the last of the Crack chicken leftovers along with the leftover broccoli.

I spent some time doing household chores and when Peter got home he grilled up some bratwurst. Once again I bugged him about including a vegetable, I cut up a cucumber, but he chose to have his meal with some spinach.

After dinner it was nice out and had cooled down so I grabbed her leash and Lexi and I took a nice walk. She was so excited to be out on a walk that we went at a pretty fast pace, and we walked for over 30 minutes.

When I got home Peter was getting ready to go to the YMCA to go swimming so I went with him and since I had already walked I did about 25 minutes on the stationary bicycle while he swam. I know I could have stayed home since I had already done exercise on my walk, but supporting each other and encouraging each other is really important, and ideally we should be doing sixty minutes of physical activity daily.

Day 93
After my morning coffee I decided to make myself some breakfast sausage. I do admit I was really craving pancakes and syrup with my sausage, but I did not have the ingredients for Keto style pancakes, nor did I have any sugar fee syrup so I guess that will have to wait for another day.

I was feeling really angry and frustrated about national political events and I just needed some escape time in the afternoon. I tried to make myself some cheese chips, but they didn't get as crunchy as I had hoped so it came out more like cheese jerky once it cooled, but it was a fun snack to eat while relaxing and reading.

After Peter got home we went out on a special date night and we both decided to not worry about staying Keto for our dinner. At first Peter said we could cheat but I challenged him and myself on that language. We were NOT cheating, we made a choice to enjoy our special meal and not worry about counting carbs. I really do believe that life is meant to be enjoyed and if I constantly focus on what I cannot have I know this 'diet' is doomed to failure. I think it is okay to make a conscious choice once in awhile to simply relax and have fun without worrying about carbs.

Peter chose a delicious looking wild boar entrée and he enjoyed it very much.

I chose to have roasted duck, and they served it with grilled parsnip, which I had never had before. It tastes like a combination of a carrot and a radish.

We both chose to share a desert, a tres leches cake and ice cream dish.

On a positive note after dinner we spent over an hour walking around the new exhibit at the Desert Botanical Garden so we did manage to get some exercise in after our meal.

Day 94 –
After my morning coffee Peter was so sweet and made me some bacon and eggs for breakfast. I had a busy day planned.

I left to go to a meeting with the local democratic office and then had to run over to my work to turn in some files. I was glad I had eaten a good breakfast because it kept me going throughout the day. I did some volunteer work in the afternoon and then when I finally got home Peter had made some Mexican style chicken casserole dish for dinner.

The only downside to really busy days is that I am not able to find time to fit exercise into my day.
In the evening I found myself feeling "snackish" so when Peter grilled himself some steaks (he made extra so he would have leftovers for the week) and they smelled so good I had to have some. I don't think I was really hungry, but it was yummy.

That 'snackish' feeling is a problem for me once in awhile. I go several days sticking with Keto and doing great, but every once in awhile I just feel hungry and I really miss having chips, crackers and other yummy snacks to eat.

As Scarlet O'Hara says – tomorrow is another day and hopefully I will feel less snackish.

Day 95 –
Peter and I got up and went to meet some friends to watch football.
The majority of items on the breakfast menu are not Keto friendly so
I simply chose to order a side of scrambled eggs and a side of bacon.
The regular entrée comes with hash browns and toast so obviously I
can't have any of those.

Later after halftime Peter ordered some wings and I had a couple
wings too as well. I drank two mimosas with very little orange juice
so I know I was still pretty low in my carbs.

In the afternoon I asked Peter to help me make the Keto cheese
crackers that I had tried before
(http://meandmychubbyadventures.blogspot.com/2018/08/our-keto-
journey-day-48.html) but this time Peter decided to fry up a couple
pieces of bacon to crumble into the crackers and we made sure to
roll them extremely thin.

They came out much better than the first time I made them, but I did
burn the edges of the first batch. I didn't mind eating the burnt one,
and they really had that crispy cracker feeling that I had been
craving.

Later for dinner Peter cooked up some mushrooms and ate them with
some leftover steak. I just had some of the leftover breakfast sausage
that I had cooked the day before.

Day 96 -
Despite not losing any weight for the past few days I am still trying
my best to stick with my new healthy eating choices. This morning I
started with some quick coffee as I ran out of the house for work.

I forgot to grab a snack and I admit that by lunchtime when we were
finished I was really hungry, but I had a few important chores to do
on the way home and I didn't get back until almost 2:00pm. I was
trying to think of a good fast lunch meal to make but realized I had

not done the dishes last night and there were no clean pans to cook with. I was tired, hungry and grumpy, so I simply grabbed some cheese and the few remaining Keto cheese crackers that peter and I had made yesterday and I ate those along with a big glass of water.

Feeling better I did the dishes and a few other important household chores and when Peter got home I decided to make myself some of the frozen shrimp with some cauliflower rice. Peter had one of his leftover steaks.

I wished that I had some other veggies to go with my meal, but it tasted great and filled me up.

After dinner Peter and I went out to a democratic meeting and on the way home we were talking about our diet. Peter was commenting that for him it is easier to see the weight loss because he holds much of his weight in his belly. He can tangibly see the results as he literally tightens his belt another notch. For me it is harder to really see results since my weight is distributed all across my body so the changes are more subtle. We both agree that we are feeling better and that is the most important part.

Day 97 -
The weather has finally cooled off so after a relaxing morning with my coffee I was able to take Lexi on a nice long walk. She was a very happy dog.

After the walk I cut up a cucumber and ate a piece of cheese.

Later in the afternoon I was feeling hungry and just couldn't decide what to eat so I made some asparagus. I roasted it in the oven with a bit of Parmesan cheese on top.

Peter called on his way home and we both decided we just didn't feel like cooking so he brought home some of the amazing cauliflower crust pizza. I do admit I had four pieces and really I should have stopped at two pieces but it was so good. The cauliflower crust has a slightly sweeter nutty flavor, but that might

just be due to the fact that we haven't really had any bread
or sugary treats for so long.

We actually looked up online and I could eat the entire pizza and
have consumed less carbs than one slice of regular pizza. A regular-
crust pizza averages 30 grams of carb per slice. That sparked a
conversation about how many carbs we used to consume without
even thinking about it. Peter and I both plan to keep with our new
low carb lifestyle even after our official 100 days have past.

Day 98 –
This morning I grabbed some coffee and headed to work. I had a
quick nut bar during my morning training and that seemed to be
enough to last until lunchtime.

Right after my morning training I had to run an errand and then I
was off to go across town to see a client for work. I had a few
minutes so I decided to stop at Wendy's and grab a quick salad for
lunch. Although the chicken did have some breading, this salad was
a good Keto choice for lunch.

When I got home I had a nice healthy snack with some cheese and
pecans. Nuts and cheese are both excellent choices for Keto, they are
higher in good fats and protein with very little carbs.

I am so happy the weather is finally cooling off, which adds a whole
bunch of great outdoor opportunities for exercise. It was so beautiful
out and Lexi politely asked me to take her on a walk, and by politely
I mean she jumped up and down and stared at me. She could feel the
beautiful weather too so we went on a really long walk that lasted for
almost two hours. Of course the one day I know I would have
exceeded my 10,000 steps I was not wearing my fitbit because I had
forgotten to put it back on after my shower. We walked a path that I
call the big loop; it is about four miles and both Lexi and I were tired
by the time we got home.

I wasn't feeling very hungry when I got home so I decided to skip
dinner and just had a couple more pieces of cheese in the evening.

Learning how to listen to my body signals is important. If I am not feeling hungry I do not need to eat. We are so trained and accustomed to eating at certain times, but our bodies may not need food at that time. Learning to listen to hunger has been one of the really important lessons of this 100-day challenge so far.

Day 99 –
It is amazing to realize we only have one more day left in our 100 day challenge.

I started my day with a nice calm morning; I had my coffee and then in mid-morning I ate some scrambled eggs and a couple pieces of bacon. I did some household chores then jumped in the shower and headed out for work.

Both work and traffic took longer than I planned but I actually wasn't too hungry. Since I have been skipping breakfast a lot, I think the bacon and eggs kept me feeling full until I got home.

For dinner I made some salmon and Peter had a steak. I also made up some oven-roasted cauliflower. I knew I was hungry because I ate really fast, which is not healthy. Eating too fast can mess with your digestion and often can make you eat more because you haven't given your body a chance to feel full yet. Another helpful hint is to make sure to drink water with your meals and take a few sips between bites.

After dinner I did treat myself to a glass of wine and one of the Atkins candy bars that Peter brought home last week. While they are not particularly healthy, they are certainly much better than a 'real' candy bar and they do help with that sweet craving that I still get once in awhile. Another thing I use when I have cravings is a spoonful of natural peanut butter. Even with low sugar, peanut butter has a sweetness that helps to curb cravings, but those carbs can add up quickly so its important to only have one or two spoons and then quickly put the jar away so you are not tempted.

100 DAYS!

Day 100 -
We did it! Peter and I made it through a full 100 days on the Keto diet and as of today I have lost 30 pounds and Peter is down 35 pounds. We both still have more to lose but this is a fantastic jump-start.

I know that the Keto diet may not be for everyone, but it really worked for us. Peter and I had a great conversation last night about our diet, what we learned during our 100 days and what our next steps will be.

The biggest lesson that we learned is that Keto does work. We were both successful at losing weight. Peter described how he thinks Keto helps get our diet back to the natural way our bodies were designed to function. I would have to agree, but for me the biggest change is avoiding the over-processed foods and empty carbs that are so prevalent today.

Another incredibly important part of the diet for us was having a partner to diet with. The ability to do this together, to encourage each other and support each other was so important to our success.

I know that people who are considering Keto will be skeptical, but if they can commit to a certain amount of time like we did they will find out that this diet does pay off.

One of the things I really enjoyed about the diet was the challenge to try out new recipes and new ways of cooking. I tend to get stuck in a rut when it comes to cooking, so this was an opportunity to try new things and we both really liked all the things we were able to eat.

I am not going to say it wasn't challenging at times. Peter said the one thing he missed the most is not having a big cold glass of milk with his meals. For me the struggle was missing the crunch of chips and crackers that I love to eat. I did find some substitutes but they really were not the same as a salty crunchy chip.

We both managed to lose a good amount of weight despite doing what I refer to as Lazy Keto. We did not carefully count macros, we simply tried each day to limit our carbs to 25 grams or less and ensure we were adding fats to our diet. Some days we were more successful than others and there were a couple times where we chose to not worry about carbs, but overall we stuck to our diet.

Now to the big question – what's next? Since we both have a large amount left to lose we are planning to continue with a low carb lifestyle. I hope to loose at least 50 more pounds and Peter has said that he wants to keep going to meet his goal as well.
We both feel healthier being on the Keto diet. I don't have that afternoon sugar crash that I used to have so often. Eating better has inspired us to be more active, which is also helping us reach our weight loss goals.

We may not be as strict about staying under 25 grams of carbs each day, but we will maintain a low carb lifestyle and if we chose to indulge on a special occasion that's okay. Feeling like I can never have a treat will cause me to fail. I love eggnog and I will chose to have a glass or two this holiday season, but I won't over-indulge and have it daily.

I won't be blogging daily but I might still do an update on our progress weekly or even monthly. I have been tracking my daily weight and I will continue to do that until I am closer to my goal weight.

We will both keep encouraging each other to exercise, it is good for us and it's a great way to spend quality time together. We both want to be around for a long time and to have the energy to play with our grandson.

Knowing that we can lose weight is incredibly motivating. It is hard work, I have to watch my portion sizes carefully to lose weight, but with all the tools and knowledge I have learned in these past 100 days, I know that I can do it.